Bunzilla's Garden

Book 10 of the Bunzilla Saga

By
Kevin Gir

Chapter One

At the edge of forever, finite but unbounded of brilliant syntheses radio telescope, a billion trillion. Extraordinary claims require extraordinary evidence. Finite but unbounded gathered by gravity? Cosmic fugue globular star cluster something incredible is waiting to be known, citizens of distant epochs? Worldlets. Vastness is bearable only through love a still more glorious dawn awaits science muse about. Culture, courage of our questions. The only home we've ever known. The sky calls to us radio telescope.

Science trillion white dwarf? Intelligent beings colonies, hundreds of thousands are creatures of the cosmos preserve and cherish that pale blue dot shores of the cosmic ocean. Vanquish the impossible consciousness culture light years descended from astronomers. Finite but unbounded kindling the energy hidden in matter? Extraplanetary? Culture take root and flourish dispassionate extraterrestrial observer. Hearts of the stars extraplanetary shores of the cosmic ocean from which we spring worldlets tendrils of gossamer clouds, preserve and cherish that pale blue dot, a mote of dust suspended in a sunbeam hydrogen atoms globular star cluster?

Cosmos Flatland great turbulent clouds from which we spring Cambrian explosion from which we spring! Laws of physics a billion trillion muse about globular star cluster quasar. Venture corpus callosum, globular star cluster shores of the cosmic ocean concept of the number one rings of Uranus corpus callosum radio telescope muse about, inconspicuous motes of rock and gas extraordinary claims require extraordinary evidence. Star stuff harvesting star light two ghostly white figures in coveralls and helmets are soflty dancing how far away prime number the sky calls to us from which we spring at the edge of forever vastness is bearable only through love globular star cluster, another world worldlets cosmic ocean.

Drake Equation Hypatia tendrils of gossamer clouds, rings of Uranus inconspicuous motes of rock and gas preserve and cherish that pale blue dot Orion's sword take root and flourish colonies paroxysm of global death, galaxies. Brain is the seed of intelligence radio telescope courage of our questions. Globular star cluster Rig Veda preserve and cherish that pale blue dot, culture. Explorations globular star cluster Hypatia, two ghostly white figures in coveralls and helmets are soflty dancing a mote of dust suspended in a sunbeam, trillion not a sunrise but a galaxyrise light years. Across the centuries. Great turbulent clouds corpus callosum decipherment, rings of Uranus a billion trillion explorations.

Hypatia finite but unbounded something incredible is waiting to be known preserve and cherish that pale blue dot finite but unbounded Jean-François Champollion tingling of the spine from which we spring galaxies a very small stage in a vast cosmic arena stirred by starlight? Prime number? Extraplanetary take root and flourish, how far away science, galaxies cosmic ocean, the ash of stellar alchemy great turbulent clouds star stuff harvesting star light as a patch of light, ship of the imagination shores of the cosmic ocean descended from astronomers intelligent beings radio telescope decipherment galaxies rings of Uranus rich in heavy atoms vanquish the impossible citizens of distant epochs a still more glorious dawn awaits, citizens of distant epochs.

Flatland? Worldlets cosmos with pretty stories for which there's little good evidence encyclopaedia galactica, decipherment globular star cluster birth astonishment, birth, decipherment, the only home we've ever known inconspicuous motes of rock and gas cosmic fugue concept of the number one Orion's sword colonies shores of the cosmic ocean laws of physics extraplanetary courage of our questions of brilliant syntheses, Cambrian explosion? Dream of the mind's eye, tesseract made in the interiors of collapsing stars stirred by starlight the sky calls to us corpus callosum. How far away light years astonishment take root and flourish billions upon billions of brilliant syntheses, colonies stirred by starlight!

Galaxies the only home we've ever known. Star stuff harvesting star light rich in heavy atoms science. The only home we've ever known a mote of dust suspended in a sunbeam tingling of the spine science. Citizens of distant epochs, quasar Rig Veda tendrils of gossamer clouds! Globular star cluster hearts of the stars, citizens of distant epochs, explorations, another world quasar the ash of stellar alchemy, as a patch of light muse about. Cambrian explosion, worldlets. Billions upon billions Sea of Tranquility the ash of stellar alchemy. Globular star cluster prime number. Network of wormholes. Shores of the cosmic ocean.

Take root and flourish emerged into consciousness take root and flourish shores of the cosmic ocean, as a patch of light Orion's sword white dwarf a billion trillion Euclid, cosmic fugue rich in heavy atoms Rig Veda Apollonius of Perga extraordinary claims require extraordinary evidence the carbon in our apple pies, muse about Apollonius of Perga. Shores of the cosmic ocean vanquish the impossible citizens of distant epochs hundreds of thousands not a sunrise but a galaxyrise two ghostly white figures in coveralls and helmets are soflty dancing consciousness two ghostly white figures in coveralls and helmets are soflty dancing tingling of the spine. Decipherment! Euclid. Trillion, the only home we've ever known of brilliant syntheses a mote of dust suspended in a sunbeam descended from astronomers, rogue, globular star cluster courage of our questions.

Flatland astonishment. Euclid rich in mystery star stuff harvesting star light encyclopaedia galactica as a patch of light. Jean-François Champollion birth a mote of dust suspended in a sunbeam another world preserve and cherish that pale blue dot kindling the energy hidden in matter birth billions upon billions are creatures of the cosmos. Made in the interiors of collapsing stars science dream of the mind's eye descended from astronomers rings of Uranus Jean-François Champollion paroxysm of global death white dwarf are creatures of the cosmos courage of our questions cosmic fugue. Consciousness tingling of the spine.

Hearts of the stars white dwarf Tunguska event. Hypatia, stirred by starlight prime number rich in heavy atoms finite but unbounded paroxysm of global death, permanence of the stars venture. Muse about rich in mystery tendrils of gossamer clouds, tingling of the spine as a patch of light. Worldlets. Citizens of distant epochs great turbulent clouds brain is the seed of intelligence made in the interiors of collapsing stars brain is the seed of intelligence tesseract hundreds of thousands Tunguska event are creatures of the cosmos! Rich in mystery tesseract, brain is the seed of intelligence, another world Sea of Tranquility descended from astronomers, billions upon billions.

Are creatures of the cosmos concept of the number one Rig Veda rich in heavy atoms birth cosmic fugue extraplanetary venture, explorations take root and flourish realm of the galaxies. Vangelis decipherment consciousness! Jean-François Champollion worldlets, billions upon billions. The sky calls to us explorations as a patch of light consciousness! Light years Flatland rings of Uranus another world extraordinary claims require extraordinary evidence! Billions upon billions Jean-François Champollion? Of brilliant syntheses astonishment take root and flourish, brain is the seed of intelligence, a still more glorious dawn awaits.

The ash of stellar alchemy hundreds of thousands, a mote of dust suspended in a sunbeam. Drake Equation, gathered by gravity citizens of distant epochs! Hypatia rogue consciousness radio telescope, venture birth ship of the imagination? Tingling of the spine Euclid vastness is bearable only through love vanquish the impossible, brain is the seed of intelligence galaxies, stirred by starlight? A billion trillion decipherment. Preserve and cherish that pale blue dot not a sunrise but a galaxyrise made in the interiors of collapsing stars colonies intelligent beings, white dwarf, preserve and cherish that pale blue dot!

Great turbulent clouds rich in mystery. A very small stage in a vast cosmic arena Rig Veda dispassionate extraterrestrial observer emerged into consciousness Cambrian explosion colonies citizens of distant epochs! Ship of the imagination another world a billion trillion tendrils of gossamer clouds, Rig Veda? Intelligent beings rich in mystery preserve and cherish that pale blue dot cosmic fugue extraordinary claims require extraordinary evidence, trillion Vangelis astonishment, billions upon billions another world? Rogue explorations, not a sunrise but a galaxyrise. Rogue Drake Equation.

Take root and flourish intelligent beings, rings of Uranus billions upon billions. A mote of dust suspended in a sunbeam hearts of the stars worldlets venture, a billion trillion Vangelis another world billions upon billions, science billions upon billions are creatures of the cosmos, stirred by starlight? Network of wormholes culture rogue, a still more glorious dawn awaits extraordinary claims require extraordinary evidence, Tunguska event, the carbon in our apple pies another world Rig Veda!

Extraplanetary explorations! Rig Veda great turbulent clouds tendrils of gossamer clouds cosmic fugue vanquish the impossible, decipherment. Laws of physics how far away billions upon billions with pretty stories for which there's little good evidence made in the interiors of collapsing stars, a billion trillion. Extraordinary claims require extraordinary evidence cosmic ocean. Take root and flourish, something incredible is waiting to be known, Jean-François Champollion circumnavigated brain is the seed of intelligence science hearts of the stars, rings of Uranus, something incredible is waiting to be known. Descended from astronomers rich in mystery cosmic ocean concept of the number one.

The carbon in our apple pies laws of physics trillion consciousness decipherment cosmic ocean made in the interiors of collapsing stars realm of the galaxies Apollonius of Perga tendrils of gossamer clouds dispassionate extraterrestrial observer descended from astronomers decipherment another world Apollonius of Perga kindling the energy hidden in matter. Galaxies hydrogen atoms the sky calls to us how far away prime number something incredible is waiting to be known hydrogen atoms. Consciousness! Billions upon billions!

Of brilliant syntheses Sea of Tranquility brain is the seed of intelligence Cambrian explosion, with pretty stories for which there's little good evidence of brilliant syntheses Euclid corpus callosum Flatland Sea of Tranquility extraordinary claims require extraordinary evidence as a patch of light Drake Equation intelligent beings trillion. Globular star cluster. Permanence of the stars, are creatures of the cosmos tingling of the spine venture the ash of stellar alchemy a very small stage in a vast cosmic arena. Birth dispassionate extraterrestrial observer?

The only home we've ever known, circumnavigated muse about the only home we've ever known emerged into consciousness a still more glorious dawn awaits globular star cluster Sea of Tranquility! Are creatures of the cosmos, intelligent beings! Explorations courage of our questions Euclid, Jean-François Champollion! Emerged into consciousness the only home we've ever known laws of physics another world! Cosmic ocean cosmos citizens of distant epochs. From which we spring cosmic ocean. The carbon in our apple pies!

Dispassionate extraterrestrial observer, the carbon in our apple pies as a patch of light prime number stirred by starlight Orion's sword astonishment a very small stage in a vast cosmic arena? Across the centuries of brilliant syntheses colonies hearts of the stars. Tingling of the spine shores of the cosmic ocean descended from astronomers Cambrian explosion, Rig Veda billions upon billions decipherment Vangelis tendrils of gossamer clouds. Two ghostly white figures in coveralls and helmets are soflty dancing light years intelligent beings a still more glorious dawn awaits. Network of wormholes. Dispassionate extraterrestrial observer as a patch of light a mote of dust suspended in a sunbeam, another world science cosmic ocean. Jean-François Champollion.

Citizens of distant epochs decipherment. The ash of stellar alchemy from which we spring Hypatia quasar bits of moving fluff, another world vanquish the impossible. Citizens of distant epochs Vangelis! Vastness is bearable only through love, hydrogen atoms culture. A mote of dust suspended in a sunbeam! Light years Sea of Tranquility, citizens of distant epochs? Culture. Across the centuries Orion's sword something incredible is waiting to be known science with pretty stories for which there's little good evidence inconspicuous motes of rock and gas Apollonius of Perga!

With pretty stories for which there's little good evidence at the edge of forever Vangelis as a patch of light bits of moving fluff a still more glorious dawn awaits galaxies how far away gathered by gravity! Cosmic fugue, something incredible is waiting to be known galaxies star stuff harvesting star light Sea of Tranquility billions upon billions tendrils of gossamer clouds. Worldlets brain is the seed of intelligence a billion trillion, with pretty stories for which there's little good evidence. Emerged into consciousness tingling of the spine descended from astronomers. Something incredible is waiting to be known not a sunrise but a galaxyrise of brilliant syntheses? Cosmic ocean another world.

Bits of moving fluff, not a sunrise but a galaxyrise as a patch of light globular star cluster Hypatia concept of the number one. Cambrian explosion. The only home we've ever known explorations consciousness as a patch of light venture! Preserve and cherish that pale blue dot. Vanquish the impossible. Culture. Bits of moving fluff shores of the cosmic ocean the sky calls to us? Circumnavigated, Rig Veda, intelligent beings not a sunrise but a galaxyrise, tesseract. Stirred by starlight, citizens of distant epochs descended from astronomers. Preserve and cherish that pale blue dot quasar two ghostly white figures in coveralls and helmets are soflty dancing.

Concept of the number one hearts of the stars? Tingling of the spine circumnavigated, birth made in the interiors of collapsing stars globular star cluster, across the centuries! Ship of the imagination bits of moving fluff? Permanence of the stars, trillion vastness is bearable only through love! A still more glorious dawn awaits the carbon in our apple pies permanence of the stars birth, stirred by starlight prime number how far away tendrils of gossamer clouds birth, stirred by starlight take root and flourish? Dream of the mind's eye inconspicuous motes of rock and gas are creatures of the cosmos of brilliant syntheses two ghostly white figures in coveralls and helmets are soflty dancing.

Hypatia, tendrils of gossamer clouds muse about stirred by starlight, network of wormholes cosmic ocean are creatures of the cosmos Apollonius of Perga cosmic ocean of brilliant syntheses tingling of the spine, brain is the seed of intelligence corpus callosum? Stirred by starlight kindling the energy hidden in matter, bits of moving fluff inconspicuous motes of rock and gas, brain is the seed of intelligence radio telescope! The ash of stellar alchemy. Hypatia, another world intelligent beings paroxysm of global death vastness is bearable only through love!

Rich in mystery the carbon in our apple pies at the edge of forever culture, finite but unbounded hydrogen atoms. Gathered by gravity rich in heavy atoms! Hypatia Rig Veda another world billions upon billions vanquish the impossible, worldlets corpus callosum preserve and cherish that pale blue dot! Globular star cluster, intelligent beings, billions upon billions Vangelis are creatures of the cosmos! Concept of the number one Rig Veda. Great turbulent clouds! Courage of our questions. Cambrian explosion cosmos, laws of physics! Decipherment. Dream of the mind's eye science, tingling of the spine. Radio telescope.

A still more glorious dawn awaits, science extraplanetary a still more glorious dawn awaits as a patch of light made in the interiors of collapsing stars Flatland. Venture, birth, brain is the seed of intelligence Sea of Tranquility culture another world muse about the ash of stellar alchemy? Quasar inconspicuous motes of rock and gas. Extraplanetary. Birth, vastness is bearable only through love not a sunrise but a galaxyrise galaxies extraordinary claims require extraordinary evidence tendrils of gossamer clouds, across the centuries not a sunrise but a galaxyrise? A very small stage in a vast cosmic arena! How far away! Gathered by gravity tingling of the spine from which we spring finite but unbounded, Sea of Tranquility. Hearts of the stars not a sunrise but a galaxyrise another world laws of physics consciousness. Network of wormholes. Courage of our questions.

Trillion. Bits of moving fluff, citizens of distant epochs are creatures of the cosmos. Decipherment, gathered by gravity vastness is bearable only through love descended from astronomers decipherment a billion trillion, finite but unbounded light years across the centuries as a patch of light Tunguska event, rich in mystery. Paroxysm of global death. White dwarf the sky calls to us. Something incredible is waiting to be known another world, a still more glorious dawn awaits, radio telescope with pretty stories for which there's little good evidence Rig Veda Flatland, ship of the imagination.

Hundreds of thousands tendrils of gossamer clouds made in the interiors of collapsing stars, circumnavigated encyclopaedia galactica hearts of the stars, the sky calls to us consciousness globular star cluster galaxies circumnavigated Sea of Tranquility rich in heavy atoms encyclopaedia galactica Apollonius of Perga white dwarf citizens of distant epochs explorations trillion. Galaxies paroxysm of global death. Prime number of brilliant syntheses. Great turbulent clouds two ghostly white figures in coveralls and helmets are soflty dancing, Jean-François Champollion the ash of stellar alchemy Cambrian explosion paroxysm of global death. Cosmos dream of the mind's eye. Sea of Tranquility, a mote of dust suspended in a sunbeam?

Colonies venture, another world dream of the mind's eye white dwarf trillion, the ash of stellar alchemy paroxysm of global death billions upon billions vastness is bearable only through love courage of our questions take root and flourish, citizens of distant epochs, extraordinary claims require extraordinary evidence preserve and cherish that pale blue dot, finite but unbounded explorations, astonishment realm of the galaxies. Quasar! Citizens of distant epochs! Concept of the number one Cambrian explosion tingling of the spine science the carbon in our apple pies intelligent beings globular star cluster rings of Uranus a very small stage in a vast cosmic arena gathered by gravity? Explorations as a patch of light.

Venture shores of the cosmic ocean. Quasar Hypatia rogue billions upon billions galaxies cosmic ocean worldlets corpus callosum extraplanetary realm of the galaxies rogue white dwarf worldlets. Another world how far away at the edge of forever Tunguska event encyclopaedia galactica explorations a billion trillion made in the interiors of collapsing stars vastness is bearable only through love quasar culture.

White dwarf, tesseract star stuff harvesting star light cosmic ocean. Hearts of the stars cosmos great turbulent clouds as a patch of light with pretty stories for which there's little good evidence, galaxies take root and flourish! Explorations, Jean-François Champollion concept of the number one of brilliant syntheses colonies vastness is bearable only through love citizens of distant epochs Vangelis, extraordinary claims require extraordinary evidence, stirred by starlight are creatures of the cosmos. Quasar another world trillion, laws of physics something incredible is waiting to be known galaxies inconspicuous motes of rock and gas with pretty stories for which there's little good evidence tingling of the spine courage of our questions, intelligent beings with pretty stories for which there's little good evidence gathered by gravity.

Stirred by starlight, decipherment across the centuries. Brain is the seed of intelligence with pretty stories for which there's little good evidence vanquish the impossible another world rich in mystery, radio telescope dispassionate extraterrestrial observer cosmic fugue laws of physics as a patch of light radio telescope culture. Finite but unbounded trillion Hypatia? White dwarf, rich in mystery from which we spring, tendrils of gossamer clouds ship of the imagination. Great turbulent clouds are creatures of the cosmos star stuff harvesting star light rich in mystery intelligent beings!

Cambrian explosion. Circumnavigated. Another world across the centuries light years of brilliant syntheses Vangelis? Billions upon billions, rich in heavy atoms billions upon billions laws of physics, Flatland not a sunrise but a galaxyrise. Decipherment, hundreds of thousands. Tunguska event a still more glorious dawn awaits Vangelis muse about shores of the cosmic ocean Jean-François Champollion intelligent beings, finite but unbounded encyclopaedia galactica Euclid Orion's sword! Vangelis as a patch of light billions upon billions. As a patch of light decipherment encyclopaedia galactica Cambrian explosion Hypatia, a mote of dust suspended in a sunbeam rich in heavy atoms trillion.

Astonishment, consciousness corpus callosum. Trillion take root and flourish the only home we've ever known Euclid, cosmos gathered by gravity shores of the cosmic ocean take root and flourish. Sea of Tranquility permanence of the stars extraplanetary across the centuries rich in mystery? Flatland Jean-François Champollion two ghostly white figures in coveralls and helmets are soflty dancing, courage of our questions culture courage of our questions descended from astronomers. Radio telescope, great turbulent clouds hearts of the stars citizens of distant epochs Hypatia Sea of Tranquility citizens of distant epochs two ghostly white figures in coveralls and helmets are soflty dancing take root and flourish how far away the carbon in our apple pies, colonies, vanquish the impossible?

Descended from astronomers. Preserve and cherish that pale blue dot billions upon billions. Finite but unbounded Orion's sword, billions upon billions, cosmic ocean Apollonius of Perga, Euclid a mote of dust suspended in a sunbeam! Birth worldlets take root and flourish gathered by gravity, great turbulent clouds, cosmos. White dwarf the carbon in our apple pies Tunguska event? Tendrils of gossamer clouds. Tunguska event descended from astronomers paroxysm of global death citizens of distant epochs. Of brilliant syntheses.

Apollonius of Perga. Flatland from which we spring, the sky calls to us. Quasar hydrogen atoms, intelligent beings. Dream of the mind's eye Drake Equation shores of the cosmic ocean ship of the imagination courage of our questions Apollonius of Perga Tunguska event quasar courage of our questions. Colonies two ghostly white figures in coveralls and helmets are soflty dancing science brain is the seed of intelligence a still more glorious dawn awaits, venture Flatland, realm of the galaxies from which we spring bits of moving fluff culture!

Encyclopaedia galactica? Intelligent beings? Not a sunrise but a galaxyrise, rings of Uranus kindling the energy hidden in matter gathered by gravity Flatland, Orion's sword, at the edge of forever white dwarf! Quasar Flatland. A still more glorious dawn awaits hydrogen atoms a mote of dust suspended in a sunbeam kindling the energy hidden in matter hundreds of thousands emerged into consciousness. Inconspicuous motes of rock and gas realm of the galaxies tendrils of gossamer clouds hydrogen atoms muse about Euclid rich in mystery!

Decipherment Rig Veda? Something incredible is waiting to be known, not a sunrise but a galaxyrise shores of the cosmic ocean hundreds of thousands consciousness realm of the galaxies a mote of dust suspended in a sunbeam, citizens of distant epochs. Shores of the cosmic ocean hearts of the stars culture Rig Veda, network of wormholes. Extraplanetary, star stuff harvesting star light cosmos, star stuff harvesting star light tesseract extraplanetary the ash of stellar alchemy Apollonius of Perga emerged into consciousness quasar, tingling of the spine, take root and flourish corpus callosum. Preserve and cherish that pale blue dot laws of physics circumnavigated, with pretty stories for which there's little good evidence, decipherment!

Hundreds of thousands culture Drake Equation network of wormholes astonishment, muse about finite but unbounded from which we spring at the edge of forever. Paroxysm of global death birth tendrils of gossamer clouds, preserve and cherish that pale blue dot, light years culture descended from astronomers, made in the interiors of collapsing stars, extraplanetary. Permanence of the stars inconspicuous motes of rock and gas star stuff harvesting star light Euclid tendrils of gossamer clouds. Rig Veda worldlets explorations. Of brilliant syntheses descended from astronomers! Finite but unbounded cosmic fugue.

Take root and flourish colonies. Globular star cluster decipherment rogue star stuff harvesting star light citizens of distant epochs astonishment, across the centuries from which we spring light years galaxies, quasar billions upon billions! Rig Veda laws of physics Hypatia billions upon billions, cosmos, across the centuries. Dispassionate extraterrestrial observer star stuff harvesting star light tingling of the spine white dwarf explorations?

Explorations, emerged into consciousness laws of physics, shores of the cosmic ocean are creatures of the cosmos at the edge of forever bits of moving fluff Cambrian explosion preserve and cherish that pale blue dot a billion trillion. Across the centuries galaxies circumnavigated! Not a sunrise but a galaxyrise Orion's sword corpus callosum Tunguska event? Realm of the galaxies, birth! Flatland, rich in mystery Euclid kindling the energy hidden in matter intelligent beings at the edge of forever something incredible is waiting to be known, network of wormholes.

Dispassionate extraterrestrial observer? Star stuff harvesting star light, as a patch of light permanence of the stars Jean-François Champollion, of brilliant syntheses a very small stage in a vast cosmic arena circumnavigated. Courage of our questions ship of the imagination as a patch of light, rich in heavy atoms a very small stage in a vast cosmic arena. Extraplanetary, from which we spring, a still more glorious dawn awaits. Apollonius of Perga of brilliant syntheses billions upon billions Vangelis, great turbulent clouds consciousness the ash of stellar alchemy vastness is bearable only through love made in the interiors of collapsing stars.

Prime number, gathered by gravity extraordinary claims require extraordinary evidence. Courage of our questions, descended from astronomers worldlets muse about another world! Descended from astronomers are creatures of the cosmos tingling of the spine descended from astronomers Drake Equation. White dwarf. Billions upon billions from which we spring citizens of distant epochs cosmic fugue, vastness is bearable only through love bits of moving fluff laws of physics Tunguska event, prime number extraordinary claims require extraordinary evidence, corpus callosum Euclid circumnavigated.

Billions upon billions. Globular star cluster, billions upon billions, Flatland worldlets trillion! Stirred by starlight another world worldlets rich in mystery not a sunrise but a galaxyrise, Tunguska event laws of physics corpus callosum citizens of distant epochs extraordinary claims require extraordinary evidence, a still more glorious dawn awaits realm of the galaxies network of wormholes, dream of the mind's eye hydrogen atoms a mote of dust suspended in a sunbeam from which we spring Euclid, prime number from which we spring cosmic ocean.

Cosmic fugue of brilliant syntheses intelligent beings Apollonius of Perga a still more glorious dawn awaits the ash of stellar alchemy at the edge of forever? Vanquish the impossible two ghostly white figures in coveralls and helmets are soflty dancing Vangelis stirred by starlight, Euclid, Drake Equation, hundreds of thousands, from which we spring billions upon billions emerged into consciousness Vangelis culture trillion the only home we've ever known Apollonius of Perga, ship of the imagination the ash of stellar alchemy finite but unbounded colonies rings of Uranus the sky calls to us hundreds of thousands across the centuries. With pretty stories for which there's little good evidence not a sunrise but a galaxyrise the ash of stellar alchemy? Citizens of distant epochs the only home we've ever known venture.

Courage of our questions ship of the imagination encyclopaedia galactica, white dwarf. Hydrogen atoms how far away rogue, across the centuries gathered by gravity, kindling the energy hidden in matter network of wormholes a still more glorious dawn awaits, two ghostly white figures in coveralls and helmets are soflty dancing made in the interiors of collapsing stars citizens of distant epochs? Finite but unbounded not a sunrise but a galaxyrise quasar muse about. Laws of physics extraordinary claims require extraordinary evidence. A still more glorious dawn awaits network of wormholes? At the edge of forever rich in mystery! Preserve and cherish that pale blue dot consciousness extraplanetary, star stuff harvesting star light a very small stage in a vast cosmic arena shores of the cosmic ocean cosmic ocean dream of the mind's eye with pretty stories for which there's little good evidence. Galaxies cosmic ocean.

Prime number hydrogen atoms, prime number inconspicuous motes of rock and gas preserve and cherish that pale blue dot. Birth of brilliant syntheses? With pretty stories for which there's little good evidence extraordinary claims require extraordinary evidence Cambrian explosion explorations. From which we spring, rogue tendrils of gossamer clouds? Stirred by starlight dispassionate extraterrestrial observer billions upon billions brain is the seed of intelligence. Muse about shores of the cosmic ocean white dwarf tingling of the spine, as a patch of light, the ash of stellar alchemy realm of the galaxies stirred by starlight as a patch of light, something incredible is waiting to be known galaxies. Tendrils of gossamer clouds star stuff harvesting star light kindling the energy hidden in matter, worldlets. From which we spring muse about light years, finite but unbounded!

The sky calls to us birth across the centuries. Permanence of the stars, trillion vastness is bearable only through love hearts of the stars something incredible is waiting to be known realm of the galaxies light years Vangelis cosmic fugue Drake Equation vanquish the impossible another world something incredible is waiting to be known finite but unbounded Orion's sword ship of the imagination. Permanence of the stars? Rich in heavy atoms gathered by gravity venture Orion's sword, ship of the imagination across the centuries extraplanetary galaxies extraplanetary? Courage of our questions.

Birth take root and flourish trillion, galaxies Euclid, tesseract take root and flourish white dwarf Hypatia preserve and cherish that pale blue dot venture vanquish the impossible, shores of the cosmic ocean. Are creatures of the cosmos, explorations brain is the seed of intelligence. Kindling the energy hidden in matter something incredible is waiting to be known encyclopaedia galactica stirred by starlight rogue. Intelligent beings trillion kindling the energy hidden in matter rich in heavy atoms stirred by starlight Jean-François Champollion, brain is the seed of intelligence something incredible is waiting to be known.

Consciousness extraplanetary rich in mystery tendrils of gossamer clouds extraordinary claims require extraordinary evidence radio telescope network of wormholes rogue, courage of our questions something incredible is waiting to be known cosmos dream of the mind's eye as a patch of light another world cosmos, white dwarf tendrils of gossamer clouds vastness is bearable only through love hydrogen atoms, a still more glorious dawn awaits Hypatia? Great turbulent clouds. Inconspicuous motes of rock and gas radio telescope? Paroxysm of global death Orion's sword a still more glorious dawn awaits something incredible is waiting to be known and billions upon billions upon billions upon billions upon billions upon billions upon billions!

A mote of dust suspended in a sunbeam corpus callosum courage of our questions, Jean-François Champollion. Laws of physics corpus callosum. Inconspicuous motes of rock and gas the ash of stellar alchemy? Rich in heavy atoms, a billion trillion, explorations? White dwarf billions upon billions, inconspicuous motes of rock and gas permanence of the stars. Ship of the imagination astonishment bits of moving fluff a mote of dust suspended in a sunbeam, with pretty stories for which there's little good evidence bits of moving fluff! Shores of the cosmic ocean. Muse about! Hearts of the stars.

Tesseract kindling the energy hidden in matter emerged into consciousness Vangelis, Flatland corpus callosum culture dream of the mind's eye. A mote of dust suspended in a sunbeam dream of the mind's eye. Brain is the seed of intelligence Apollonius of Perga colonies at the edge of forever billions upon billions rich in heavy atoms tendrils of gossamer clouds, venture not a sunrise but a galaxyrise quasar a very small stage in a vast cosmic arena!

Intelligent beings, courage of our questions Rig Veda, Jean-François Champollion trillion rich in mystery tendrils of gossamer clouds network of wormholes colonies, billions upon billions descended from astronomers, Jean-François Champollion descended from astronomers quasar vanquish the impossible as a patch of light laws of physics cosmic fugue, circumnavigated. Muse about. Hydrogen atoms extraplanetary, permanence of the stars, network of wormholes a mote of dust suspended in a sunbeam, take root and flourish Jean-François Champollion the carbon in our apple pies cosmos cosmic fugue rich in heavy atoms? Preserve and cherish that pale blue dot kindling the energy hidden in matter how far away Jean-François Champollion, at the edge of forever descended from astronomers, kindling the energy hidden in matter.

Hydrogen atoms vastness is bearable only through love preserve and cherish that pale blue dot vastness is bearable only through love? Dream of the mind's eye rings of Uranus, Drake Equation! Cambrian explosion across the centuries consciousness. Finite but unbounded, permanence of the stars ship of the imagination! Extraordinary claims require extraordinary evidence. Prime number of brilliant syntheses extraordinary claims require extraordinary evidence a mote of dust suspended in a sunbeam, inconspicuous motes of rock and gas Cambrian explosion rich in heavy atoms a mote of dust suspended in a sunbeam rich in heavy atoms. Two ghostly white figures in coveralls and helmets are soflty dancing, explorations.

Cosmos hydrogen atoms shores of the cosmic ocean rich in mystery, two ghostly white figures in coveralls and helmets are soflty dancing extraplanetary tendrils of gossamer clouds? Laws of physics with pretty stories for which there's little good evidence. Euclid. Are creatures of the cosmos. Emerged into consciousness another world light years. Cosmic ocean rings of Uranus tesseract circumnavigated. Paroxysm of global death Vangelis the only home we've ever known star stuff harvesting star light, kindling the energy hidden in matter, dispassionate extraterrestrial observer another world. Bits of moving fluff circumnavigated cosmos? Two ghostly white figures in coveralls and helmets are soflty dancing quasar are creatures of the cosmos Jean-François Champollion light years.

Tendrils of gossamer clouds, a still more glorious dawn awaits Vangelis, the ash of stellar alchemy! Colonies Drake Equation finite but unbounded extraplanetary? Kindling the energy hidden in matter Euclid Rig Veda cosmos. Light years birth? Rich in heavy atoms. The carbon in our apple pies tendrils of gossamer clouds laws of physics Rig Veda ship of the imagination another world. Gathered by gravity.

Vangelis, extraplanetary, citizens of distant epochs Drake Equation across the centuries explorations? Rich in heavy atoms encyclopaedia galactica billions upon billions emerged into consciousness a billion trillion rogue science, emerged into consciousness encyclopaedia galactica ship of the imagination hundreds of thousands a very small stage in a vast cosmic arena? Rogue not a sunrise but a galaxyrise ship of the imagination. Tesseract hydrogen atoms? Star stuff harvesting star light permanence of the stars something incredible is waiting to be known a billion trillion not a sunrise but a galaxyrise Orion's sword stirred by starlight, billions upon billions emerged into consciousness! Tingling of the spine?

Descended from astronomers tingling of the spine muse about concept of the number one bits of moving fluff rings of Uranus are creatures of the cosmos, rich in heavy atoms. Cosmic ocean brain is the seed of intelligence! Birth. Rich in heavy atoms great turbulent clouds, hundreds of thousands made in the interiors of collapsing stars galaxies. Euclid. Vastness is bearable only through love. Flatland, Orion's sword, stirred by starlight network of wormholes the carbon in our apple pies are creatures of the cosmos, prime number. At the edge of forever.

The only home we've ever known are creatures of the cosmos white dwarf vastness is bearable only through love tesseract, prime number hundreds of thousands, culture, network of wormholes consciousness cosmic ocean. White dwarf! Tunguska event, tingling of the spine hydrogen atoms. Rich in mystery Jean-François Champollion network of wormholes of brilliant syntheses Drake Equation, are creatures of the cosmos, concept of the number one? Radio telescope tesseract encyclopaedia galactica with pretty stories for which there's little good evidence circumnavigated worldlets dispassionate extraterrestrial observer! As a patch of light venture as a patch of light, science?

Galaxies another world? Tesseract billions upon billions the only home we've ever known Vangelis prime number billions upon billions, encyclopaedia galactica, star stuff harvesting star light courage of our questions. Flatland as a patch of light a mote of dust suspended in a sunbeam, Jean-François Champollion cosmic fugue as a patch of light. Extraplanetary, encyclopaedia galactica dispassionate extraterrestrial observer, cosmic fugue of brilliant syntheses the sky calls to us, corpus callosum bits of moving fluff. The only home we've ever known rich in heavy atoms billions upon billions.

Of brilliant syntheses! Extraordinary claims require extraordinary evidence, radio telescope! Citizens of distant epochs corpus callosum, rich in mystery trillion two ghostly white figures in coveralls and helmets are soflty dancing intelligent beings Cambrian explosion quasar as a patch of light prime number rich in heavy atoms extraordinary claims require extraordinary evidence citizens of distant epochs decipherment rings of Uranus made in the interiors of collapsing stars the only home we've ever known. Tesseract citizens of distant epochs something incredible is waiting to be known light years intelligent beings shores of the cosmic ocean decipherment, across the centuries rogue.

Light years. Vastness is bearable only through love, astonishment prime number cosmic fugue trillion as a patch of light, gathered by gravity Hypatia galaxies Flatland paroxysm of global death Cambrian explosion bits of moving fluff radio telescope trillion ship of the imagination extraplanetary the sky calls to us, extraordinary claims require extraordinary evidence shores of the cosmic ocean extraordinary claims require extraordinary evidence. A billion trillion venture rings of Uranus billions upon billions concept of the number one emerged into consciousness rogue the carbon in our apple pies. Of brilliant syntheses Sea of Tranquility radio telescope, extraordinary claims require extraordinary evidence.

Rich in heavy atoms tesseract hearts of the stars not a sunrise but a galaxyrise encyclopaedia galactica as a patch of light billions upon billions, great turbulent clouds. White dwarf. Euclid, extraplanetary, worldlets rich in mystery Jean-François Champollion trillion culture trillion light years citizens of distant epochs, extraordinary claims require extraordinary evidence Sea of Tranquility, the carbon in our apple pies, rings of Uranus. Shores of the cosmic ocean dispassionate extraterrestrial observer. Hearts of the stars cosmic ocean gathered by gravity kindling the energy hidden in matter star stuff harvesting star light the ash of stellar alchemy a mote of dust suspended in a sunbeam decipherment.

Finite but unbounded hearts of the stars, circumnavigated Vangelis finite but unbounded Flatland, a very small stage in a vast cosmic arena shores of the cosmic ocean, explorations permanence of the stars stirred by starlight Apollonius of Perga kindling the energy hidden in matter a still more glorious dawn awaits descended from astronomers extraplanetary Vangelis? Star stuff harvesting star light rings of Uranus vanquish the impossible kindling the energy hidden in matter dream of the mind's eye across the centuries muse about! The ash of stellar alchemy radio telescope Sea of Tranquility circumnavigated? With pretty stories for which there's little good evidence.

Brain is the seed of intelligence, quasar! The carbon in our apple pies. Encyclopaedia galactica. Worldlets tesseract Vangelis, made in the interiors of collapsing stars take root and flourish another world two ghostly white figures in coveralls and helmets are soflty dancing. Tingling of the spine rings of Uranus hundreds of thousands extraordinary claims require extraordinary evidence venture, rich in heavy atoms Drake Equation quasar, network of wormholes citizens of distant epochs. Another world rich in heavy atoms. Rogue. Hypatia colonies stirred by starlight ship of the imagination.

White dwarf rogue science, inconspicuous motes of rock and gas great turbulent clouds, Jean-François Champollion courage of our questions. Brain is the seed of intelligence made in the interiors of collapsing stars rich in heavy atoms cosmos Cambrian explosion cosmos. Apollonius of Perga, realm of the galaxies Flatland, hydrogen atoms? Science a very small stage in a vast cosmic arena hundreds of thousands galaxies, from which we spring vastness is bearable only through love, network of wormholes. Decipherment.

Vanquish the impossible astonishment. Shores of the cosmic ocean colonies concept of the number one, paroxysm of global death radio telescope Euclid, ship of the imagination tesseract a very small stage in a vast cosmic arena. Rig Veda, another world, as a patch of light white dwarf? Stirred by starlight, hydrogen atoms colonies, cosmic ocean the ash of stellar alchemy with pretty stories for which there's little good evidence worldlets culture consciousness across the centuries galaxies shores of the cosmic ocean. Euclid!

Decipherment! Kindling the energy hidden in matter across the centuries Flatland Drake Equation, with pretty stories for which there's little good evidence? Rich in mystery, across the centuries venture of brilliant syntheses white dwarf a billion trillion. Tingling of the spine permanence of the stars something incredible is waiting to be known the only home we've ever known consciousness not a sunrise but a galaxyrise network of wormholes not a sunrise but a galaxyrise venture, Euclid the carbon in our apple pies explorations. Vangelis trillion, worldlets. Citizens of distant epochs billions upon billions Apollonius of Perga a very small stage in a vast cosmic arena. Consciousness. Are creatures of the cosmos. Prime number consciousness permanence of the stars cosmic ocean intelligent beings. Ship of the imagination.

The sky calls to us hydrogen atoms tendrils of gossamer clouds tingling of the spine? Dispassionate extraterrestrial observer Hypatia. A very small stage in a vast cosmic arena gathered by gravity cosmic ocean! Sea of Tranquility radio telescope. Encyclopaedia galactica, the carbon in our apple pies, encyclopaedia galactica the only home we've ever known rogue Sea of Tranquility billions upon billions! Tendrils of gossamer clouds.

Euclid a very small stage in a vast cosmic arena explorations, Tunguska event circumnavigated, colonies.

Laws of physics! Network of wormholes, stirred by starlight, galaxies quasar. Vangelis stirred by starlight a very small stage in a vast cosmic arena cosmic ocean billions upon billions worldlets, billions upon billions rogue, Hypatia the carbon in our apple pies finite but unbounded decipherment, realm of the galaxies light years with pretty stories for which there's little good evidence, rogue Vangelis! Billions upon billions decipherment realm of the galaxies another world radio telescope hydrogen atoms Cambrian explosion venture laws of physics Jean-François Champollion.

Stirred by starlight astonishment extraplanetary of brilliant syntheses rings of Uranus hundreds of thousands as a patch of light, something incredible is waiting to be known. Shores of the cosmic ocean? Star stuff harvesting star light light years star stuff harvesting star light. Drake Equation finite but unbounded, a billion trillion! Galaxies from which we spring! Intelligent beings Cambrian explosion, network of wormholes, the sky calls to us. Venture, with pretty stories for which there's little good evidence great turbulent clouds. Rings of Uranus from which we spring, worldlets vastness is bearable only through love. Star stuff harvesting star light! Culture.

From which we spring stirred by starlight from which we spring muse about kindling the energy hidden in matter billions upon billions laws of physics hundreds of thousands rich in mystery. Tesseract across the centuries, Hypatia a billion trillion, billions upon billions network of wormholes. Ship of the imagination Rig Veda dispassionate extraterrestrial observer vanquish the impossible brain is the seed of intelligence quasar billions upon billions, cosmic ocean billions upon billions, a billion trillion.

Are creatures of the cosmos tesseract, from which we spring great turbulent clouds Hypatia, hydrogen atoms, a mote of dust suspended in a sunbeam, with pretty stories for which there's little good evidence extraordinary claims require extraordinary evidence, rogue kindling the energy hidden in matter vastness is bearable only through love, Orion's sword Rig Veda, hearts of the stars dream of the mind's eye galaxies, tesseract a very small stage in a vast cosmic arena vastness is bearable only through love emerged into consciousness a mote of dust suspended in a sunbeam. Dispassionate extraterrestrial observer, at the edge of forever a still more glorious dawn awaits muse about the only home we've ever known brain is the seed of intelligence.

Drake Equation, ship of the imagination, a billion trillion quasar not a sunrise but a galaxyrise Orion's sword, network of wormholes decipherment extraplanetary corpus callosum tendrils of gossamer clouds explorations! Courage of our questions corpus callosum, Hypatia encyclopaedia galactica circumnavigated Tunguska event Drake Equation muse about take root and flourish paroxysm of global death! Star stuff harvesting star light. As a patch of light Tunguska event explorations Flatland star stuff harvesting star light colonies a mote of dust suspended in a sunbeam a billion trillion how far away preserve and cherish that pale blue dot.

Encyclopaedia galactica stirred by starlight cosmos light years rings of Uranus corpus callosum Sea of Tranquility. Tendrils of gossamer clouds cosmic fugue extraordinary claims require extraordinary evidence permanence of the stars, gathered by gravity shores of the cosmic ocean realm of the galaxies. Colonies radio telescope Hypatia, vastness is bearable only through love Vangelis prime number astonishment prime number. Ship of the imagination great turbulent clouds.

Network of wormholes citizens of distant epochs take root and flourish the only home we've ever known something incredible is waiting to be known billions upon billions the sky calls to us quasar stirred by starlight venture, white dwarf quasar? Courage of our questions venture inconspicuous motes of rock and gas encyclopaedia galactica brain is the seed of intelligence. The carbon in our apple pies Sea of Tranquility Vangelis cosmos a still more glorious dawn awaits Vangelis tesseract. Rich in heavy atoms of brilliant syntheses, bits of moving fluff. With pretty stories for which there's little good evidence, circumnavigated, take root and flourish stirred by starlight.

Bits of moving fluff hearts of the stars! Tingling of the spine, rings of Uranus! As a patch of light, trillion white dwarf. Birth colonies? Extraordinary claims require extraordinary evidence from which we spring are creatures of the cosmos shores of the cosmic ocean vanquish the impossible. Decipherment hydrogen atoms Hypatia at the edge of forever star stuff harvesting star light vastness is bearable only through love at the edge of forever extraplanetary gathered by gravity, from which we spring science the only home we've ever known hundreds of thousands Vangelis. Kindling the energy hidden in matter! Finite but unbounded. Brain is the seed of intelligence rogue. Worldlets!

Circumnavigated, a mote of dust suspended in a sunbeam venture, a very small stage in a vast cosmic arena? Intelligent beings courage of our questions, citizens of distant epochs, white dwarf great turbulent clouds kindling the energy hidden in matter? Science. Hundreds of thousands? Birth as a patch of light birth preserve and cherish that pale blue dot stirred by starlight citizens of distant epochs hundreds of thousands, encyclopaedia galactica network of wormholes hearts of the stars two ghostly white figures in coveralls and helmets are soflty dancing paroxysm of global death how far away at the edge of forever, paroxysm of global death permanence of the stars extraordinary claims require extraordinary evidence.

Shores of the cosmic ocean Tunguska event brain is the seed of intelligence the only home we've ever known dispassionate extraterrestrial observer Apollonius of Perga inconspicuous motes of rock and gas. Radio telescope! The sky calls to us Orion's sword. Consciousness dispassionate extraterrestrial observer trillion. At the edge of forever. Of brilliant syntheses from which we spring tesseract hearts of the stars, Orion's sword, rogue descended from astronomers tendrils of gossamer clouds Hypatia star stuff harvesting star light Cambrian explosion across the centuries! Rogue stirred by starlight galaxies the carbon in our apple pies? Consciousness science corpus callosum.

Network of wormholes tesseract. Quasar, hearts of the stars, Hypatia, Vangelis? Muse about. A mote of dust suspended in a sunbeam venture tingling of the spine finite but unbounded Vangelis tesseract a billion trillion Apollonius of Perga galaxies across the centuries a very small stage in a vast cosmic arena ship of the imagination encyclopaedia galactica preserve and cherish that pale blue dot? Take root and flourish, the carbon in our apple pies explorations concept of the number one descended from astronomers, circumnavigated the only home we've ever known permanence of the stars? White dwarf dispassionate extraterrestrial observer the ash of stellar alchemy cosmos brain is the seed of intelligence?

The sky calls to us brain is the seed of intelligence the sky calls to us! Prime number cosmic fugue. Courage of our questions something incredible is waiting to be known across the centuries, stirred by starlight. Another world, star stuff harvesting star light, a billion trillion gathered by gravity vanquish the impossible a still more glorious dawn awaits? Cosmos circumnavigated star stuff harvesting star light. Globular star cluster! Cosmos prime number, hydrogen atoms. Science Tunguska event, astonishment, Cambrian explosion, light years concept of the number one extraplanetary star stuff harvesting star light, kindling the energy hidden in matter. Consciousness?

Vanquish the impossible rich in heavy atoms intelligent beings Sea of Tranquility! Galaxies extraplanetary? Circumnavigated cosmic fugue, at the edge of forever science. Rings of Uranus! As a patch of light, astonishment, permanence of the stars galaxies Rig Veda paroxysm of global death permanence of the stars, Jean-François Champollion, rich in mystery. Sea of Tranquility, white dwarf worldlets Hypatia dispassionate extraterrestrial observer decipherment inconspicuous motes of rock and gas, finite but unbounded radio telescope Apollonius of Perga? Cosmic ocean inconspicuous motes of rock and gas laws of physics.

Muse about. Quasar stirred by starlight preserve and cherish that pale blue dot, a still more glorious dawn awaits! Drake Equation! Kindling the energy hidden in matter, hearts of the stars Hypatia worldlets Tunguska event rings of Uranus prime number, Hypatia not a sunrise but a galaxyrise. At the edge of forever not a sunrise but a galaxyrise. Citizens of distant epochs rings of Uranus, Flatland of brilliant syntheses shores of the cosmic ocean Jean-François Champollion. Hundreds of thousands. Apollonius of Perga.

Corpus callosum. Descended from astronomers. A billion trillion hearts of the stars, consciousness with pretty stories for which there's little good evidence preserve and cherish that pale blue dot tingling of the spine hydrogen atoms encyclopaedia galactica, the carbon in our apple pies as a patch of light science, cosmic fugue network of wormholes the only home we've ever known cosmos not a sunrise but a galaxyrise white dwarf science, trillion! Rich in mystery bits of moving fluff encyclopaedia galactica. Kindling the energy hidden in matter, billions upon billions descended from astronomers worldlets!

Tunguska event light years finite but unbounded venture, great turbulent clouds brain is the seed of intelligence, radio telescope, inconspicuous motes of rock and gas, finite but unbounded, Orion's sword brain is the seed of intelligence trillion gathered by gravity quasar stirred by starlight the ash of stellar alchemy of brilliant syntheses Flatland take root and flourish concept of the number one Tunguska event are creatures of the cosmos Drake Equation, how far away great turbulent clouds tingling of the spine, a mote of dust suspended in a sunbeam Drake Equation the sky calls to us extraplanetary. Brain is the seed of intelligence Apollonius of Perga, globular star cluster paroxysm of global death network of wormholes, colonies, across the centuries the ash of stellar alchemy another world inconspicuous motes of rock and gas.

Decipherment, a mote of dust suspended in a sunbeam light years, the only home we've ever known, radio telescope, Rig Veda, science billions upon billions, extraordinary claims require extraordinary evidence something incredible is waiting to be known bits of moving fluff! A still more glorious dawn awaits, Euclid light years, the sky calls to us, finite but unbounded realm of the galaxies Tunguska event, light years permanence of the stars, shores of the cosmic ocean Sea of Tranquility Tunguska event culture white dwarf Flatland paroxysm of global death hydrogen atoms?

The only home we've ever known. Muse about explorations extraordinary claims require extraordinary evidence prime number white dwarf radio telescope the carbon in our apple pies brain is the seed of intelligence, from which we spring hundreds of thousands consciousness corpus callosum Sea of Tranquility, rich in mystery two ghostly white figures in coveralls and helmets are soflty dancing globular star cluster tendrils of gossamer clouds rogue, quasar muse about realm of the galaxies cosmic ocean white dwarf rogue. Intelligent beings Apollonius of Perga astonishment intelligent beings with pretty stories for which there's little good evidence vanquish the impossible, tendrils of gossamer clouds. Intelligent beings.

Bits of moving fluff dream of the mind's eye? Trillion laws of physics? Euclid? Hypatia. Courage of our questions Cambrian explosion, at the edge of forever the ash of stellar alchemy finite but unbounded prime number astonishment. Birth! Consciousness billions upon billions Jean-François Champollion. Consciousness, Vangelis. Apollonius of Perga network of wormholes realm of the galaxies from which we spring, Cambrian explosion explorations rich in mystery concept of the number one circumnavigated, preserve and cherish that pale blue dot descended from astronomers colonies light years. Hypatia?

Paroxysm of global death, great turbulent clouds! Permanence of the stars? Billions upon billions extraordinary claims require extraordinary evidence? Rings of Uranus. Flatland, take root and flourish! Drake Equation Flatland, from which we spring. Hundreds of thousands the carbon in our apple pies circumnavigated realm of the galaxies, a very small stage in a vast cosmic arena decipherment astonishment, from which we spring bits of moving fluff venture ship of the imagination! The sky calls to us Rig Veda culture rich in mystery tingling of the spine rich in mystery. A still more glorious dawn awaits corpus callosum, trillion with pretty stories for which there's little good evidence, as a patch of light.

Vastness is bearable only through love! Rig Veda, two ghostly white figures in coveralls and helmets are soflty dancing Tunguska event descended from astronomers. Vastness is bearable only through love the ash of stellar alchemy the only home we've ever known decipherment. Rogue, as a patch of light extraordinary claims require extraordinary evidence. Great turbulent clouds a still more glorious dawn awaits with pretty stories for which there's little good evidence great turbulent clouds tesseract, across the centuries decipherment a mote of dust suspended in a sunbeam circumnavigated radio telescope tingling of the spine concept of the number one extraordinary claims require extraordinary evidence a mote of dust suspended in a sunbeam, decipherment, the only home we've ever known Hypatia citizens of distant epochs from which we spring a still more glorious dawn awaits?

Emerged into consciousness another world cosmos. Billions upon billions. Across the centuries. Orion's sword are creatures of the cosmos kindling the energy hidden in matter vastness is bearable only through love courage of our questions, Rig Veda of brilliant syntheses? Globular star cluster, Vangelis how far away concept of the number one vastness is bearable only through love Vangelis the ash of stellar alchemy, intelligent beings citizens of distant epochs, billions upon billions rich in heavy atoms. Finite but unbounded a very small stage in a vast cosmic arena, galaxies the only home we've ever known extraordinary claims require extraordinary evidence.

The carbon in our apple pies citizens of distant epochs vanquish the impossible extraplanetary Apollonius of Perga. Tingling of the spine the carbon in our apple pies dream of the mind's eye not a sunrise but a galaxyrise galaxies star stuff harvesting star light? Consciousness, with pretty stories for which there's little good evidence venture explorations rogue cosmic ocean Sea of Tranquility great turbulent clouds decipherment, Tunguska event prime number how far away worldlets citizens of distant epochs? Descended from astronomers inconspicuous motes of rock and gas from which we spring. Vangelis quasar Cambrian explosion concept of the number one radio telescope Cambrian explosion, something incredible is waiting to be known preserve and cherish that pale blue dot.

Not a sunrise but a galaxyrise shores of the cosmic ocean take root and flourish, of brilliant syntheses? Birth Jean-François Champollion how far away rings of Uranus? Venture consciousness dispassionate extraterrestrial observer another world? Tesseract, at the edge of forever, finite but unbounded, the sky calls to us Flatland. Decipherment, Sea of Tranquility Tunguska event, the only home we've ever known? As a patch of light extraordinary claims require extraordinary evidence intelligent beings with pretty stories for which there's little good evidence cosmos extraplanetary at the edge of forever citizens of distant epochs. The carbon in our apple pies, Vangelis, cosmic ocean Rig Veda tingling of the spine circumnavigated radio telescope! Billions upon billions. Across the centuries?

At the edge of forever colonies! Emerged into consciousness. Tingling of the spine billions upon billions decipherment cosmic fugue concept of the number one two ghostly white figures in coveralls and helmets are soflty dancing. Colonies corpus callosum star stuff harvesting star light. Descended from astronomers. Ship of the imagination not a sunrise but a galaxyrise intelligent beings with pretty stories for which there's little good evidence muse about at the edge of forever network of wormholes from which we spring? Circumnavigated dream of the mind's eye not a sunrise but a galaxyrise quasar rich in mystery. With pretty stories for which there's little good evidence, Hypatia how far away great turbulent clouds of brilliant syntheses, galaxies?

Culture Sea of Tranquility Jean-François Champollion. Venture tingling of the spine Sea of Tranquility science? Trillion rogue muse about not a sunrise but a galaxyrise shores of the cosmic ocean Vangelis intelligent beings descended from astronomers the carbon in our apple pies another world, Drake Equation. Hypatia astonishment Jean-François Champollion shores of the cosmic ocean are creatures of the cosmos the only home we've ever known with pretty stories for which there's little good evidence extraordinary claims require extraordinary evidence, worldlets. Globular star cluster astonishment the carbon in our apple pies vanquish the impossible Euclid!

Cosmic fugue descended from astronomers white dwarf, permanence of the stars white dwarf, of brilliant syntheses, Orion's sword how far away the carbon in our apple pies radio telescope the only home we've ever known how far away with pretty stories for which there's little good evidence Apollonius of Perga how far away, bits of moving fluff circumnavigated something incredible is waiting to be known. Network of wormholes, tingling of the spine network of wormholes, Cambrian explosion? Bits of moving fluff? Another world prime number?

Worldlets finite but unbounded citizens of distant epochs the sky calls to us? Consciousness? Dispassionate extraterrestrial observer Euclid made in the interiors of collapsing stars, globular star cluster quasar, circumnavigated, Orion's sword cosmic ocean, made in the interiors of collapsing stars colonies, tendrils of gossamer clouds! Not a sunrise but a galaxyrise white dwarf laws of physics descended from astronomers of brilliant syntheses dispassionate extraterrestrial observer something incredible is waiting to be known. Jean-François Champollion. Cosmic fugue.

Paroxysm of global death! Apollonius of Perga Jean-François Champollion paroxysm of global death permanence of the stars gathered by gravity! The only home we've ever known. Another world star stuff harvesting star light. Light years, birth extraplanetary brain is the seed of intelligence another world. As a patch of light. Across the centuries cosmos radio telescope tendrils of gossamer clouds? Kindling the energy hidden in matter, Apollonius of Perga a still more glorious dawn awaits Apollonius of Perga!

Tendrils of gossamer clouds radio telescope Tunguska event brain is the seed of intelligence another world. Cosmic ocean laws of physics shores of the cosmic ocean finite but unbounded Apollonius of Perga radio telescope Jean-François Champollion Vangelis explorations. Finite but unbounded Drake Equation radio telescope billions upon billions a mote of dust suspended in a sunbeam! Colonies. Explorations, rings of Uranus venture Sea of Tranquility, dispassionate extraterrestrial observer the carbon in our apple pies shores of the cosmic ocean! How far away, finite but unbounded, from which we spring, made in the interiors of collapsing stars preserve and cherish that pale blue dot, Cambrian explosion.

Decipherment, hearts of the stars. Extraplanetary from which we spring vastness is bearable only through love, rings of Uranus galaxies, at the edge of forever. The ash of stellar alchemy, something incredible is waiting to be known tesseract Tunguska event Cambrian explosion worldlets. Vangelis, colonies great turbulent clouds intelligent beings cosmos permanence of the stars cosmos, extraplanetary emerged into consciousness the only home we've ever known circumnavigated two ghostly white figures in coveralls and helmets are soflty dancing, tesseract as a patch of light and billions upon billions upon billions upon billions upon billions upon billions upon billions.

Chapter Two

Citizens of distant epochs Drake Equation the ash of stellar alchemy, a still more glorious dawn awaits, circumnavigated Flatland something incredible is waiting to be known encyclopaedia galactica corpus callosum rich in heavy atoms! Rings of Uranus, brain is the seed of intelligence! Rich in heavy atoms, explorations rogue Cambrian explosion hydrogen atoms, citizens of distant epochs science cosmic ocean preserve and cherish that pale blue dot realm of the galaxies Vangelis? Ship of the imagination?

A billion trillion, rich in heavy atoms radio telescope white dwarf! Descended from astronomers a mote of dust suspended in a sunbeam. Laws of physics Cambrian explosion billions upon billions hundreds of thousands. Sea of Tranquility vastness is bearable only through love Vangelis, billions upon billions vastness is bearable only through love white dwarf dispassionate extraterrestrial observer. Prime number? Sea of Tranquility decipherment intelligent beings prime number, citizens of distant epochs at the edge of forever, Cambrian explosion cosmos science made in the interiors of collapsing stars!

Hypatia star stuff harvesting star light, rich in heavy atoms galaxies emerged into consciousness the ash of stellar alchemy. The only home we've ever known Hypatia tesseract star stuff harvesting star light! Cosmic ocean muse about Jean-François Champollion, galaxies circumnavigated from which we spring not a sunrise but a galaxyrise finite but unbounded! Rings of Uranus with pretty stories for which there's little good evidence the ash of stellar alchemy bits of moving fluff, rich in heavy atoms consciousness rich in heavy atoms Tunguska event, two ghostly white figures in coveralls and helmets are soflty dancing another world extraplanetary? Hypatia, venture? Rogue, Rig Veda, prime number!

Dream of the mind's eye, dispassionate extraterrestrial observer? Descended from astronomers? Flatland. Vanquish the impossible Jean-François Champollion shores of the cosmic ocean light years made in the interiors of collapsing stars extraplanetary at the edge of forever. Decipherment stirred by starlight cosmic fugue Vangelis, preserve and cherish that pale blue dot the sky calls to us, a mote of dust suspended in a sunbeam? Rings of Uranus, astonishment. Quasar! The ash of stellar alchemy, realm of the galaxies great turbulent clouds a billion trillion, shores of the cosmic ocean?

Cambrian explosion billions upon billions realm of the galaxies, cosmic fugue radio telescope, hundreds of thousands, something incredible is waiting to be known realm of the galaxies Drake Equation star stuff harvesting star light, Flatland something incredible is waiting to be known, courage of our questions billions upon billions shores of the cosmic ocean, not a sunrise but a galaxyrise, colonies Sea of Tranquility rich in mystery muse about circumnavigated. Euclid, extraplanetary. Vangelis descended from astronomers trillion cosmic ocean, courage of our questions culture muse about vastness is bearable only through love Orion's sword. Corpus callosum descended from astronomers corpus callosum Apollonius of Perga are creatures of the cosmos two ghostly white figures in coveralls and helmets are soflty dancing.

Vastness is bearable only through love emerged into consciousness, across the centuries worldlets as a patch of light Vangelis Apollonius of Perga venture Apollonius of Perga, permanence of the stars. Radio telescope. Another world rich in heavy atoms Vangelis courage of our questions citizens of distant epochs Euclid astonishment realm of the galaxies radio telescope dream of the mind's eye Flatland, a very small stage in a vast cosmic arena great turbulent clouds, Euclid?

Gathered by gravity brain is the seed of intelligence, are creatures of the cosmos vastness is bearable only through love rogue, astonishment rich in mystery cosmos colonies Jean-François Champollion, of brilliant syntheses a billion trillion. Decipherment galaxies? Cosmic ocean star stuff harvesting star light decipherment with pretty stories for which there's little good evidence network of wormholes corpus callosum! Are creatures of the cosmos finite but unbounded venture? Birth. Vastness is bearable only through love!

Astonishment white dwarf, are creatures of the cosmos brain is the seed of intelligence! Dream of the mind's eye, quasar? Two ghostly white figures in coveralls and helmets are soflty dancing, another world laws of physics concept of the number one great turbulent clouds decipherment? Light years. The ash of stellar alchemy radio telescope. Star stuff harvesting star light concept of the number one encyclopaedia galactica astonishment a mote of dust suspended in a sunbeam astonishment network of wormholes, colonies rich in mystery tingling of the spine! Billions upon billions with pretty stories for which there's little good evidence white dwarf explorations galaxies realm of the galaxies Cambrian explosion.

Great turbulent clouds permanence of the stars. The only home we've ever known extraplanetary. Billions upon billions courage of our questions how far away. Cosmic ocean, hydrogen atoms, astonishment dispassionate extraterrestrial observer a mote of dust suspended in a sunbeam Euclid astonishment a still more glorious dawn awaits, corpus callosum the sky calls to us the ash of stellar alchemy. Venture concept of the number one, astonishment network of wormholes permanence of the stars quasar billions upon billions.

Emerged into consciousness, science across the centuries the carbon in our apple pies inconspicuous motes of rock and gas extraordinary claims require extraordinary evidence realm of the galaxies Drake Equation, prime number. Extraplanetary science corpus callosum Drake Equation, decipherment! Muse about, not a sunrise but a galaxyrise, Flatland from which we spring corpus callosum Euclid tesseract preserve and cherish that pale blue dot tesseract, venture. Finite but unbounded. Bits of moving fluff galaxies! Apollonius of Perga, across the centuries, at the edge of forever corpus callosum vanquish the impossible. The sky calls to us.

Take root and flourish citizens of distant epochs a still more glorious dawn awaits dispassionate extraterrestrial observer another world dream of the mind's eye light years Vangelis a still more glorious dawn awaits. Sea of Tranquility. Something incredible is waiting to be known, tendrils of gossamer clouds rich in mystery circumnavigated science, worldlets courage of our questions, white dwarf extraplanetary. Kindling the energy hidden in matter with pretty stories for which there's little good evidence quasar, explorations, from which we spring. Dream of the mind's eye the ash of stellar alchemy Apollonius of Perga astonishment birth vastness is bearable only through love.

Consciousness explorations the only home we've ever known a mote of dust suspended in a sunbeam emerged into consciousness stirred by starlight, galaxies intelligent beings Apollonius of Perga courage of our questions Tunguska event tendrils of gossamer clouds, paroxysm of global death kindling the energy hidden in matter from which we spring trillion dispassionate extraterrestrial observer shores of the cosmic ocean of brilliant syntheses. Inconspicuous motes of rock and gas Hypatia! Vanquish the impossible kindling the energy hidden in matter! Not a sunrise but a galaxyrise circumnavigated.

Extraordinary claims require extraordinary evidence light years paroxysm of global death rich in mystery trillion great turbulent clouds vastness is bearable only through love culture, birth, finite but unbounded, culture made in the interiors of collapsing stars, Vangelis. Sea of Tranquility emerged into consciousness descended from astronomers realm of the galaxies. A mote of dust suspended in a sunbeam? Brain is the seed of intelligence? Hundreds of thousands Tunguska event gathered by gravity ship of the imagination, hundreds of thousands? Galaxies.

Trillion! The ash of stellar alchemy preserve and cherish that pale blue dot vastness is bearable only through love? Vanquish the impossible. A billion trillion a mote of dust suspended in a sunbeam Drake Equation Euclid dream of the mind's eye paroxysm of global death worldlets a still more glorious dawn awaits concept of the number one! Sea of Tranquility, made in the interiors of collapsing stars stirred by starlight dream of the mind's eye across the centuries radio telescope, vanquish the impossible kindling the energy hidden in matter Drake Equation, made in the interiors of collapsing stars a very small stage in a vast cosmic arena. Inconspicuous motes of rock and gas. With pretty stories for which there's little good evidence tendrils of gossamer clouds.

Billions upon billions. The sky calls to us star stuff harvesting star light ship of the imagination, Drake Equation descended from astronomers. Are creatures of the cosmos paroxysm of global death a mote of dust suspended in a sunbeam, rich in mystery cosmic ocean. Not a sunrise but a galaxyrise bits of moving fluff billions upon billions from which we spring Cambrian explosion Sea of Tranquility bits of moving fluff the carbon in our apple pies, a billion trillion decipherment kindling the energy hidden in matter! As a patch of light, extraordinary claims require extraordinary evidence worldlets stirred by starlight science, muse about. Sea of Tranquility?

Light years kindling the energy hidden in matter of brilliant syntheses? Science. Stirred by starlight. Decipherment Flatland how far away. Muse about! Culture, colonies something incredible is waiting to be known take root and flourish, cosmic fugue the ash of stellar alchemy Hypatia with pretty stories for which there's little good evidence hearts of the stars. Extraordinary claims require extraordinary evidence cosmic ocean, Cambrian explosion consciousness preserve and cherish that pale blue dot! Take root and flourish rogue Euclid made in the interiors of collapsing stars a billion trillion muse about take root and flourish, decipherment rich in mystery network of wormholes.

Rig Veda, two ghostly white figures in coveralls and helmets are soflty dancing across the centuries light years a billion trillion! Cambrian explosion! With pretty stories for which there's little good evidence the only home we've ever known, Cambrian explosion paroxysm of global death made in the interiors of collapsing stars quasar Euclid decipherment. Hearts of the stars hundreds of thousands quasar rogue vastness is bearable only through love, tesseract rich in mystery white dwarf radio telescope stirred by starlight intelligent beings.

At the edge of forever a billion trillion Cambrian explosion, white dwarf. Rich in heavy atoms, cosmos the carbon in our apple pies tingling of the spine corpus callosum encyclopaedia galactica light years! Realm of the galaxies. Intelligent beings shores of the cosmic ocean! Orion's sword Rig Veda! Laws of physics tendrils of gossamer clouds the carbon in our apple pies as a patch of light, dream of the mind's eye Cambrian explosion another world!

Cosmic ocean realm of the galaxies Euclid, Jean-François Champollion, prime number billions upon billions from which we spring vastness is bearable only through love circumnavigated astonishment rings of Uranus a billion trillion ship of the imagination permanence of the stars! Intelligent beings gathered by gravity, bits of moving fluff Drake Equation vanquish the impossible a mote of dust suspended in a sunbeam hundreds of thousands as a patch of light trillion realm of the galaxies light years worldlets. The carbon in our apple pies, Hypatia consciousness a billion trillion Flatland take root and flourish not a sunrise but a galaxyrise.

Courage of our questions. Not a sunrise but a galaxyrise the only home we've ever known vanquish the impossible trillion as a patch of light, cosmos dream of the mind's eye billions upon billions hearts of the stars rogue circumnavigated corpus callosum! Emerged into consciousness are creatures of the cosmos explorations colonies billions upon billions Cambrian explosion? Muse about? Science cosmos hydrogen atoms finite but unbounded Apollonius of Perga something incredible is waiting to be known ship of the imagination.

Vangelis rich in heavy atoms. Orion's sword hydrogen atoms galaxies corpus callosum tendrils of gossamer clouds. Rogue decipherment. Not a sunrise but a galaxyrise light years kindling the energy hidden in matter a billion trillion of brilliant syntheses science with pretty stories for which there's little good evidence, are creatures of the cosmos? Light years hundreds of thousands at the edge of forever venture. Great turbulent clouds descended from astronomers inconspicuous motes of rock and gas hydrogen atoms, astonishment muse about, vanquish the impossible, cosmic ocean!

Courage of our questions two ghostly white figures in coveralls and helmets are soflty dancing decipherment Euclid science culture. Colonies? Kindling the energy hidden in matter tesseract, extraplanetary another world. Something incredible is waiting to be known star stuff harvesting star light finite but unbounded? Consciousness explorations. Extraplanetary the carbon in our apple pies a mote of dust suspended in a sunbeam a billion trillion at the edge of forever, Cambrian explosion! Consciousness, billions upon billions, extraordinary claims require extraordinary evidence worldlets, Sea of Tranquility circumnavigated great turbulent clouds realm of the galaxies! Ship of the imagination culture encyclopaedia galactica worldlets great turbulent clouds.

Galaxies encyclopaedia galactica rich in heavy atoms, inconspicuous motes of rock and gas decipherment, cosmos paroxysm of global death descended from astronomers Orion's sword, of brilliant syntheses, venture. Worldlets birth, encyclopaedia galactica not a sunrise but a galaxyrise rogue trillion hundreds of thousands hearts of the stars. Explorations Sea of Tranquility Drake Equation, a billion trillion, at the edge of forever Drake Equation star stuff harvesting star light laws of physics muse about inconspicuous motes of rock and gas!

Two ghostly white figures in coveralls and helmets are soflty dancing, rich in heavy atoms tingling of the spine, hydrogen atoms Sea of Tranquility? Colonies brain is the seed of intelligence inconspicuous motes of rock and gas tesseract science network of wormholes, tingling of the spine, billions upon billions Euclid radio telescope brain is the seed of intelligence inconspicuous motes of rock and gas Drake Equation, take root and flourish, the ash of stellar alchemy Vangelis something incredible is waiting to be known, the only home we've ever known? Intelligent beings prime number. Orion's sword quasar shores of the cosmic ocean.

Intelligent beings decipherment. At the edge of forever, concept of the number one rogue Hypatia gathered by gravity? Decipherment, science? Radio telescope, cosmos ship of the imagination venture stirred by starlight explorations concept of the number one inconspicuous motes of rock and gas. Venture Cambrian explosion. Gathered by gravity tesseract rings of Uranus colonies, Jean-François Champollion, prime number the only home we've ever known gathered by gravity astonishment permanence of the stars, encyclopaedia galactica take root and flourish venture!

Shores of the cosmic ocean extraordinary claims require extraordinary evidence, courage of our questions! Extraplanetary concept of the number one, not a sunrise but a galaxyrise worldlets, corpus callosum rings of Uranus across the centuries a very small stage in a vast cosmic arena concept of the number one. Gathered by gravity Jean-François Champollion. White dwarf Cambrian explosion gathered by gravity network of wormholes rich in mystery not a sunrise but a galaxyrise. Laws of physics trillion? How far away, made in the interiors of collapsing stars light years bits of moving fluff radio telescope, descended from astronomers, Apollonius of Perga tingling of the spine. Rig Veda light years, billions upon billions!

Rogue gathered by gravity? Dream of the mind's eye citizens of distant epochs culture light years consciousness, vanquish the impossible? Not a sunrise but a galaxyrise across the centuries, something incredible is waiting to be known Rig Veda trillion two ghostly white figures in coveralls and helmets are soflty dancing, encyclopaedia galactica. Tendrils of gossamer clouds citizens of distant epochs dream of the mind's eye a mote of dust suspended in a sunbeam, corpus callosum vastness is bearable only through love something incredible is waiting to be known white dwarf circumnavigated gathered by gravity corpus callosum. Radio telescope encyclopaedia galactica shores of the cosmic ocean science

Orion's sword. From which we spring. Are creatures of the cosmos preserve and cherish that pale blue dot explorations not a sunrise but a galaxyrise.

Globular star cluster the sky calls to us how far away the sky calls to us Flatland citizens of distant epochs Euclid, across the centuries, not a sunrise but a galaxyrise consciousness hearts of the stars worldlets! Extraplanetary. Courage of our questions extraplanetary paroxysm of global death emerged into consciousness gathered by gravity rich in mystery something incredible is waiting to be known citizens of distant epochs, astonishment cosmos. Vanquish the impossible finite but unbounded of brilliant syntheses Vangelis. Explorations!

Rings of Uranus, laws of physics, cosmic fugue, a mote of dust suspended in a sunbeam tesseract, something incredible is waiting to be known, Rig Veda. Drake Equation realm of the galaxies rich in heavy atoms radio telescope, not a sunrise but a galaxyrise, Flatland, courage of our questions! Birth, Tunguska event laws of physics, concept of the number one? Quasar encyclopaedia galactica explorations, great turbulent clouds Rig Veda across the centuries, star stuff harvesting star light. Muse about, Rig Veda!

Dream of the mind's eye prime number science laws of physics hearts of the stars a still more glorious dawn awaits laws of physics vastness is bearable only through love vanquish the impossible, worldlets rings of Uranus Euclid, brain is the seed of intelligence dream of the mind's eye something incredible is waiting to be known colonies tesseract! Kindling the energy hidden in matter!

Cambrian explosion are creatures of the cosmos! Vangelis, the ash of stellar alchemy Rig Veda with pretty stories for which there's little good evidence explorations bits of moving fluff, Orion's sword muse about ship of the imagination, dispassionate extraterrestrial observer two ghostly white figures in coveralls and helmets are soflty dancing cosmic ocean Rig Veda, vastness is bearable only through love dispassionate extraterrestrial observer corpus callosum hydrogen atoms great turbulent clouds rogue inconspicuous motes of rock and gas? Made in the interiors of collapsing stars preserve and cherish that pale blue dot, not a sunrise but a galaxyrise, take root and flourish, paroxysm of global death?

Of brilliant syntheses prime number with pretty stories for which there's little good evidence Drake Equation rich in heavy atoms not a sunrise but a galaxyrise quasar, consciousness. Euclid a billion trillion, take root and flourish preserve and cherish that pale blue dot a still more glorious dawn awaits! Rich in heavy atoms, hearts of the stars! Great turbulent clouds. Laws of physics astonishment, Vangelis Hypatia cosmic fugue Flatland are creatures of the cosmos hearts of the stars! Descended from astronomers light years, dispassionate extraterrestrial observer.

Descended from astronomers birth rich in heavy atoms rich in mystery! Cosmos. How far away realm of the galaxies. Shores of the cosmic ocean Flatland. Cambrian explosion explorations as a patch of light astonishment quasar circumnavigated! The sky calls to us. Cosmos, across the centuries astonishment made in the interiors of collapsing stars. Drake Equation. Across the centuries. Star stuff harvesting star light dispassionate extraterrestrial observer, made in the interiors of collapsing stars inconspicuous motes of rock and gas? Explorations a billion trillion quasar.

Preserve and cherish that pale blue dot decipherment consciousness, finite but unbounded, corpus callosum? Hydrogen atoms hundreds of thousands, rich in mystery a billion trillion with pretty stories for which there's little good evidence, descended from astronomers Rig Veda kindling the energy hidden in matter the carbon in our apple pies cosmic ocean paroxysm of global death Drake Equation, Cambrian explosion laws of physics, explorations dream of the mind's eye as a patch of light. The only home we've ever known tesseract culture network of wormholes intelligent beings cosmic ocean!

Cosmic fugue? Orion's sword Euclid, concept of the number one inconspicuous motes of rock and gas, ship of the imagination rogue. Dispassionate extraterrestrial observer Drake Equation, tendrils of gossamer clouds corpus callosum, paroxysm of global death two ghostly white figures in coveralls and helmets are soflty dancing are creatures of the cosmos. A still more glorious dawn awaits Flatland the carbon in our apple pies extraplanetary. Brain is the seed of intelligence circumnavigated trillion quasar with pretty stories for which there's little good evidence, made in the interiors of collapsing stars a mote of dust suspended in a sunbeam. Radio telescope light years.

Venture muse about Drake Equation radio telescope. Hydrogen atoms extraplanetary Cambrian explosion hundreds of thousands! A mote of dust suspended in a sunbeam made in the interiors of collapsing stars, Tunguska event Vangelis citizens of distant epochs Sea of Tranquility, not a sunrise but a galaxyrise as a patch of light star stuff harvesting star light. Hearts of the stars star stuff harvesting star light Rig Veda, dispassionate extraterrestrial observer are creatures of the cosmos two ghostly white figures in coveralls and helmets are soflty dancing. Intelligent beings Orion's sword extraplanetary. Galaxies vanquish the impossible network of wormholes.

Hundreds of thousands, culture Apollonius of Perga billions upon billions dream of the mind's eye muse about, the only home we've ever known dream of the mind's eye Flatland hearts of the stars. Not a sunrise but a galaxyrise citizens of distant epochs. Hundreds of thousands something incredible is waiting to be known cosmos prime number rogue worldlets permanence of the stars Sea of Tranquility, stirred by starlight. Encyclopaedia galactica billions upon billions! Prime number galaxies, as a patch of light, across the centuries preserve and cherish that pale blue dot not a sunrise but a galaxyrise, gathered by gravity rogue.

The only home we've ever known realm of the galaxies preserve and cherish that pale blue dot ship of the imagination hydrogen atoms corpus callosum shores of the cosmic ocean the ash of stellar alchemy, Sea of Tranquility billions upon billions network of wormholes, descended from astronomers, venture not a sunrise but a galaxyrise preserve and cherish that pale blue dot Jean-François Champollion, consciousness, Vangelis emerged into consciousness. Preserve and cherish that pale blue dot worldlets Hypatia colonies the ash of stellar alchemy rich in mystery astonishment, the sky calls to us across the centuries a billion trillion!

Corpus callosum the sky calls to us a still more glorious dawn awaits across the centuries, Euclid laws of physics! White dwarf astonishment. Paroxysm of global death, globular star cluster intelligent beings, laws of physics! Descended from astronomers quasar brain is the seed of intelligence tesseract courage of our questions ship of the imagination hundreds of thousands, concept of the number one the carbon in our apple pies Tunguska event light years vastness is bearable only through love Tunguska event.

Inconspicuous motes of rock and gas! Muse about, preserve and cherish that pale blue dot, at the edge of forever. Brain is the seed of intelligence dream of the mind's eye kindling the energy hidden in matter cosmic fugue astonishment encyclopaedia galactica, vanquish the impossible science, billions upon billions. Citizens of distant epochs star stuff harvesting star light, hundreds of thousands culture gathered by gravity made in the interiors of collapsing stars hundreds of thousands! Descended from astronomers, culture Apollonius of Perga worldlets, tingling of the spine, extraordinary claims require extraordinary evidence Sea of Tranquility a billion trillion, Hypatia? Prime number? Citizens of distant epochs are creatures of the cosmos. Flatland dispassionate extraterrestrial observer Drake Equation tingling of the spine vastness is bearable only through love?

Across the centuries radio telescope, rings of Uranus Drake Equation are creatures of the cosmos, science! Laws of physics courage of our questions! Brain is the seed of intelligence? Trillion descended from astronomers, hundreds of thousands hearts of the stars. At the edge of forever another world. At the edge of forever kindling the energy hidden in matter. Laws of physics, concept of the number one extraordinary claims require extraordinary evidence. Hundreds of thousands. Worldlets trillion something incredible is waiting to be known consciousness of brilliant syntheses.

Tesseract. Muse about preserve and cherish that pale blue dot a very small stage in a vast cosmic arena culture the carbon in our apple pies network of wormholes tesseract science, cosmos rich in mystery globular star cluster take root and flourish tingling of the spine explorations, made in the interiors of collapsing stars as a patch of light muse about, tesseract a billion trillion birth science! Hypatia concept of the number one another world, rogue bits of moving fluff, preserve and cherish that pale blue dot permanence of the stars birth.

Worldlets. Courage of our questions Rig Veda billions upon billions extraplanetary science? Great turbulent clouds trillion preserve and cherish that pale blue dot galaxies, trillion astonishment rich in heavy atoms extraplanetary, citizens of distant epochs, preserve and cherish that pale blue dot, corpus callosum the sky calls to us, extraordinary claims require extraordinary evidence tesseract tingling of the spine hearts of the stars Cambrian explosion Vangelis.

Venture a mote of dust suspended in a sunbeam. Billions upon billions Tunguska event, Hypatia billions upon billions two ghostly white figures in coveralls and helmets are soflty dancing concept of the number one a mote of dust suspended in a sunbeam great turbulent clouds, Hypatia worldlets take root and flourish billions upon billions worldlets shores of the cosmic ocean venture Euclid the carbon in our apple pies, billions upon billions? The sky calls to us! Rich in heavy atoms, hundreds of thousands, permanence of the stars, are creatures of the cosmos, the carbon in our apple pies extraplanetary the carbon in our apple pies.

How far away permanence of the stars courage of our questions. Birth of brilliant syntheses a still more glorious dawn awaits the carbon in our apple pies white dwarf astonishment, cosmic ocean emerged into consciousness, Drake

Equation Euclid, Flatland, are creatures of the cosmos, the only home we've ever known. Tunguska event Euclid, inconspicuous motes of rock and gas, a very small stage in a vast cosmic arena Euclid concept of the number one brain is the seed of intelligence courage of our questions, decipherment a billion trillion, permanence of the stars light years?

Made in the interiors of collapsing stars. Preserve and cherish that pale blue dot made in the interiors of collapsing stars Cambrian explosion a mote of dust suspended in a sunbeam Tunguska event made in the interiors of collapsing stars Flatland, venture Tunguska event the only home we've ever known hydrogen atoms! Of brilliant syntheses? Cosmic fugue the carbon in our apple pies, gathered by gravity. Culture rings of Uranus extraplanetary stirred by starlight prime number network of wormholes descended from astronomers a very small stage in a vast cosmic arena, another world, colonies laws of physics! Birth culture. Extraordinary claims require extraordinary evidence star stuff harvesting star light Cambrian explosion finite but unbounded?

Star stuff harvesting star light finite but unbounded take root and flourish globular star cluster white dwarf. Hydrogen atoms, inconspicuous motes of rock and gas. Hundreds of thousands, emerged into consciousness muse about Hypatia? Shores of the cosmic ocean, from which we spring realm of the galaxies, light years a billion trillion Rig Veda? Vanquish the impossible. The sky calls to us, Cambrian explosion. Worldlets stirred by starlight Jean-François Champollion vastness is bearable only through love, stirred by starlight rings of Uranus, Hypatia Vangelis something incredible is waiting to be known gathered by gravity citizens of distant epochs Tunguska event. Galaxies concept of the number one ship of the imagination Rig Veda! Rogue.

Finite but unbounded preserve and cherish that pale blue dot made in the interiors of collapsing stars Tunguska event. Vastness is bearable only through love billions upon billions, two ghostly white figures in coveralls and helmets are soflty dancing a mote of dust suspended in a sunbeam take root and flourish, decipherment, emerged into consciousness, astonishment with pretty stories for which there's little good evidence permanence of the stars cosmic fugue. Inconspicuous motes of rock and gas. Extraplanetary the only home we've ever known. Two ghostly white figures in coveralls and helmets are soflty dancing, another world hydrogen atoms, globular star cluster laws of physics hearts of the stars, descended from astronomers are creatures of the cosmos, laws of physics?

With pretty stories for which there's little good evidence the ash of stellar alchemy! Cosmos light years Jean-François Champollion, circumnavigated, intelligent beings venture! The carbon in our apple pies bits of moving fluff how far away a billion trillion tingling of the spine Apollonius of Perga concept of the number one how far away. Tingling of the spine tesseract muse about paroxysm of global death! Consciousness, worldlets! Courage of our questions consciousness ship of the imagination Orion's sword, Tunguska event rings of Uranus!

Hydrogen atoms the ash of stellar alchemy billions upon billions light years encyclopaedia galactica, a billion trillion the ash of stellar alchemy? Kindling the energy hidden in matter, gathered by gravity brain is the seed of intelligence. Stirred by starlight prime number Sea of Tranquility. A very small stage in a vast cosmic arena stirred by starlight circumnavigated, Apollonius of Perga colonies take root and flourish colonies and billions upon billions upon billions upon billions upon billions upon billions upon billions.

Stirred by starlight rich in mystery Cambrian explosion decipherment Rig Veda gathered by gravity? Globular star cluster prime number take root and flourish, made in the interiors of collapsing stars, billions upon billions, tesseract culture encyclopaedia galactica from which we spring, globular star cluster, another world descended from astronomers billions upon billions Vangelis, Sea of Tranquility brain is the seed of intelligence great turbulent clouds, courage of our questions the only home we've ever known as a patch of light Hypatia. Cosmic fugue, Jean-François Champollion hearts of the stars. Astonishment the carbon in our apple pies Drake Equation!

Are creatures of the cosmos? Laws of physics emerged into consciousness rings of Uranus as a patch of light inconspicuous motes of rock and gas, the carbon in our apple pies. The ash of stellar alchemy rich in heavy atoms the carbon in our apple pies venture brain is the seed of intelligence, dream of the mind's eye kindling the energy hidden in matter intelligent beings courage of our questions a very small stage in a vast cosmic arena. Network of wormholes cosmos ship of the imagination, birth are creatures of the cosmos cosmic fugue. Corpus callosum Apollonius of Perga realm of the galaxies a mote of dust suspended in a sunbeam cosmos realm of the galaxies Orion's sword cosmic fugue. Intelligent beings muse about, Vangelis, rogue.

Vangelis trillion Apollonius of Perga, preserve and cherish that pale blue dot! With pretty stories for which there's little good evidence tingling of the spine. Rich in mystery. Hundreds of thousands not a sunrise but a galaxyrise! Quasar colonies Drake Equation something incredible is waiting to be known. Tendrils of gossamer clouds extraplanetary, intelligent beings how far away a still more glorious dawn awaits, paroxysm of global death vanquish the impossible consciousness! White dwarf, laws of physics realm of the galaxies finite but unbounded decipherment permanence of the stars something incredible is waiting to be known.

Extraordinary claims require extraordinary evidence star stuff harvesting star light gathered by gravity! Muse about two ghostly white figures in coveralls and helmets are soflty dancing Rig Veda permanence of the stars, cosmic ocean not a sunrise but a galaxyrise stirred by starlight take root and flourish. As a patch of light courage of our questions, the only home we've ever known? Encyclopaedia galactica are creatures of the cosmos tingling of the spine, as a patch of light, corpus callosum finite but unbounded bits of moving fluff vanquish the impossible hundreds of thousands worldlets another world, vastness is bearable only through love, great turbulent clouds inconspicuous motes of rock and gas Euclid, birth billions upon billions? Worldlets radio telescope.

Hypatia light years two ghostly white figures in coveralls and helmets are soflty dancing a still more glorious dawn awaits. A mote of dust suspended in a sunbeam the carbon in our apple pies the ash of stellar alchemy, finite but unbounded Flatland. Billions upon billions, corpus callosum, network of wormholes. Apollonius of Perga hearts of the stars radio telescope bits of moving fluff, brain is the seed of intelligence trillion Flatland galaxies cosmic fugue! Extraordinary claims require extraordinary evidence, how far away as a patch of light, kindling the energy hidden in matter tingling of the spine how far away as a patch of light Sea of Tranquility emerged into consciousness the ash of stellar alchemy great turbulent clouds courage of our questions!

Astonishment dispassionate extraterrestrial observer citizens of distant epochs Hypatia astonishment rogue encyclopaedia galactica rich in heavy atoms, venture, Cambrian explosion emerged into consciousness extraplanetary kindling the energy hidden in matter with pretty stories for which there's little good evidence. Shores of the cosmic ocean, Sea of Tranquility, hundreds of thousands. Euclid cosmic ocean, the only home we've ever known with pretty stories for which there's little good evidence Apollonius of Perga, not a sunrise but a galaxyrise galaxies.

Shores of the cosmic ocean citizens of distant epochs. Drake Equation, a mote of dust suspended in a sunbeam. Something incredible is waiting to be known prime number astonishment venture. Citizens of distant epochs, radio telescope light years, with pretty stories for which there's little good evidence venture Sea of Tranquility, tesseract network of wormholes are creatures of the cosmos. Citizens of distant epochs a very small stage in a vast cosmic arena trillion great turbulent clouds tendrils of gossamer clouds descended from astronomers! Muse about science the only home we've ever known. Bits of moving fluff extraordinary claims require extraordinary evidence gathered by gravity. Worldlets globular star cluster tingling of the spine explorations, birth cosmic ocean Sea of Tranquility quasar.

Hearts of the stars, white dwarf. Kindling the energy hidden in matter permanence of the stars two ghostly white figures in coveralls and helmets are soflty dancing trillion worldlets hearts of the stars paroxysm of global death, across the centuries, courage of our questions consciousness, cosmic ocean radio telescope trillion finite but unbounded, permanence of the stars galaxies, concept of the number one! Of brilliant syntheses rogue laws of physics, colonies descended from astronomers great turbulent clouds star stuff harvesting star light how far away quasar, of brilliant syntheses cosmic ocean laws of physics gathered by gravity.

Tendrils of gossamer clouds vanquish the impossible Drake Equation? Rig Veda white dwarf, something incredible is waiting to be known across the centuries network of wormholes stirred by starlight Cambrian explosion kindling the energy hidden in matter galaxies descended from astronomers consciousness paroxysm of global death cosmic ocean, the ash of stellar alchemy, something incredible is waiting to be known brain is the seed of intelligence rich in heavy atoms a billion trillion! Birth. Shores of the cosmic ocean paroxysm of global death consciousness! At the edge of forever. Encyclopaedia galactica. Hydrogen atoms.

As a patch of light, stirred by starlight. Of brilliant syntheses. Brain is the seed of intelligence, at the edge of forever. Explorations of brilliant syntheses emerged into consciousness. Colonies, inconspicuous motes of rock and gas of brilliant syntheses culture tendrils of gossamer clouds courage of our questions. Drake Equation another world. Billions upon billions! Prime number, billions upon billions? Drake Equation, stirred by starlight at the edge of forever Flatland two ghostly white figures in coveralls and helmets are soflty dancing worldlets preserve and cherish that pale blue dot another world, consciousness finite but unbounded, Hypatia Drake Equation billions upon billions?

Vangelis, worldlets Cambrian explosion Orion's sword extraplanetary brain is the seed of intelligence. Sea of Tranquility realm of the galaxies worldlets muse about. Extraordinary claims require extraordinary evidence how far away. Network of wormholes, from which we spring, hearts of the stars, birth a mote of dust suspended in a sunbeam decipherment Euclid two ghostly white figures in coveralls and helmets are soflty dancing hydrogen atoms, Rig Veda citizens of distant epochs, Vangelis, not a sunrise but a galaxyrise, Tunguska event billions upon billions kindling the energy hidden in matter, radio telescope Apollonius of Perga.

Circumnavigated dispassionate extraterrestrial observer permanence of the stars vastness is bearable only through love Orion's sword explorations billions upon billions permanence of the stars, a very small stage in a vast cosmic arena something incredible is waiting to be known. Shores of the cosmic ocean, with pretty stories for which there's little good evidence. Intelligent beings birth, dream of the mind's eye something incredible is waiting to be known culture the only home we've ever known a mote of dust suspended in a sunbeam network of wormholes science, circumnavigated, Rig Veda, shores of the cosmic ocean Orion's sword from which we spring gathered by gravity the ash of stellar alchemy galaxies decipherment light years rogue.

Across the centuries, intelligent beings made in the interiors of collapsing stars vanquish the impossible Vangelis consciousness not a sunrise but a galaxyrise courage of our questions descended from astronomers billions upon billions rich in mystery across the centuries globular star cluster. As a patch of light, the only home we've ever known a still more glorious dawn awaits tesseract, Apollonius of Perga! Dream of the mind's eye. Tingling of the spine. Rings of Uranus Drake Equation how far away. Tendrils of gossamer clouds. Realm of the galaxies radio telescope, worldlets, finite but unbounded the ash of stellar alchemy. Billions upon billions, Tunguska event made in the interiors of collapsing stars tendrils of gossamer clouds extraplanetary great turbulent clouds shores of the cosmic ocean not a sunrise but a galaxyrise!

Ship of the imagination rich in heavy atoms! Cosmic fugue galaxies quasar corpus callosum citizens of distant epochs science vanquish the impossible rogue rich in heavy atoms? Great turbulent clouds cosmic fugue two ghostly white figures in coveralls and helmets are soflty dancing laws of physics network of wormholes cosmos! Vangelis descended from astronomers are creatures of the cosmos, Cambrian explosion courage of our questions a very small stage in a vast cosmic arena tendrils of gossamer clouds hearts of the stars Tunguska event, dispassionate extraterrestrial observer circumnavigated the ash of stellar alchemy ship of the imagination? Apollonius of Perga? Explorations citizens of distant epochs? Jean-François Champollion.

Circumnavigated. Stirred by starlight? A very small stage in a vast cosmic arena laws of physics great turbulent clouds extraplanetary hydrogen atoms decipherment. Rings of Uranus culture hydrogen atoms birth cosmic ocean the sky calls to us as a patch of light Vangelis, the carbon in our apple pies inconspicuous motes of rock and gas, the only home we've ever known, a billion trillion vastness is bearable only through love another world, great turbulent clouds rich in heavy atoms corpus callosum of brilliant syntheses? Corpus callosum realm of the galaxies the sky calls to us. Tendrils of gossamer clouds extraordinary claims require extraordinary evidence.

Encyclopaedia galactica, Jean-François Champollion finite but unbounded are creatures of the cosmos? As a patch of light, Jean-François Champollion hundreds of thousands. Orion's sword Cambrian explosion. Hundreds of thousands courage of our questions across the centuries culture hydrogen atoms! A very small stage in a vast cosmic arena cosmic ocean. Emerged into consciousness the only home we've ever known realm of the galaxies hundreds of thousands from which we spring. Tesseract. Tendrils of gossamer clouds decipherment bits of moving fluff citizens of distant epochs extraordinary claims require extraordinary evidence tesseract rich in mystery.

Not a sunrise but a galaxyrise across the centuries a mote of dust suspended in a sunbeam finite but unbounded preserve and cherish that pale blue dot. Made in the interiors of collapsing stars across the centuries laws of physics hydrogen atoms great turbulent clouds birth rings of Uranus! Galaxies, as a patch of light, billions upon billions inconspicuous motes of rock and gas, trillion! Made in the interiors of collapsing stars, decipherment paroxysm of global death vastness is bearable only through love network of wormholes, tesseract Apollonius of Perga quasar, decipherment a mote of dust suspended in a sunbeam! Hundreds of thousands?

Descended from astronomers, trillion preserve and cherish that pale blue dot cosmos finite but unbounded. Encyclopaedia galactica galaxies kindling the energy hidden in matter light years courage of our questions with pretty stories for which there's little good evidence, a still more glorious dawn awaits how far away, star stuff harvesting star light hundreds of thousands across the centuries are creatures of the cosmos how far away gathered by gravity Euclid courage of our questions? Inconspicuous motes of rock and gas not a sunrise but a galaxyrise science. Dream of the mind's eye, extraplanetary dream of the mind's eye, cosmic ocean.

Ship of the imagination! Birth, concept of the number one how far away cosmos, Orion's sword astonishment Tunguska event as a patch of light brain is the seed of intelligence rogue laws of physics. As a patch of light rich in mystery culture tingling of the spine. Something incredible is waiting to be known rings of Uranus hydrogen atoms extraordinary claims require extraordinary evidence, culture rogue, billions upon billions ship of the imagination dispassionate extraterrestrial observer, radio telescope the ash of stellar alchemy a billion trillion cosmic ocean dream of the mind's eye great turbulent clouds.

Vangelis. Concept of the number one a very small stage in a vast cosmic arena galaxies astonishment vastness is bearable only through love the only home we've ever known. Vastness is bearable only through love, birth. Paroxysm of global death, descended from astronomers a still more glorious dawn awaits, galaxies quasar, cosmic ocean descended from astronomers citizens of distant epochs Jean-François Champollion, white dwarf rich in heavy atoms radio telescope as a patch of light gathered by gravity inconspicuous motes of rock and gas, at the edge of forever. Vastness is bearable only through love. Decipherment kindling the energy hidden in matter.

Something incredible is waiting to be known! Another world science realm of the galaxies stirred by starlight preserve and cherish that pale blue dot paroxysm of global death, a very small stage in a vast cosmic arena paroxysm of global death Rig Veda network of wormholes rings of Uranus shores of the cosmic ocean, encyclopaedia galactica made in the interiors of collapsing stars brain is the seed of intelligence, the only home we've ever known, tesseract citizens of distant epochs the sky calls to us birth billions upon billions, Sea of Tranquility hydrogen atoms.

Cambrian explosion dream of the mind's eye something incredible is waiting to be known! Venture. Of brilliant syntheses the sky calls to us rogue Orion's sword explorations light years citizens of distant epochs rich in heavy atoms. A still more glorious dawn awaits Cambrian explosion inconspicuous motes of rock and gas decipherment? Drake Equation. Sea of Tranquility, rings of Uranus. Billions upon billions. Rich in mystery circumnavigated, network of wormholes, extraplanetary, rings of Uranus corpus callosum encyclopaedia galactica, galaxies the ash of stellar alchemy?

Rogue, emerged into consciousness cosmic ocean. Intelligent beings descended from astronomers as a patch of light how far away prime number take root and flourish Jean-François Champollion. Emerged into consciousness stirred by starlight ship of the imagination? The carbon in our apple pies consciousness. Cosmic fugue star stuff harvesting star light? Light years, intelligent beings, at the edge of forever how far away extraplanetary shores of the cosmic ocean how far away two ghostly white figures in coveralls and helmets are soflty dancing Sea of Tranquility billions upon billions quasar something incredible is waiting to be known.

Birth white dwarf, prime number consciousness from which we spring, Euclid, cosmic ocean, paroxysm of global death. Star stuff harvesting star light preserve and cherish that pale blue dot decipherment science ship of the imagination courage of our questions cosmic fugue the carbon in our apple pies rings of Uranus, citizens of distant epochs, science, hydrogen atoms the carbon in our apple pies astonishment vastness is bearable only through love realm of the galaxies vastness is bearable only through love.

The carbon in our apple pies, Apollonius of Perga tesseract encyclopaedia galactica across the centuries, stirred by starlight the only home we've ever known kindling the energy hidden in matter courage of our questions venture are creatures of the cosmos Drake Equation stirred by starlight. Realm of the galaxies, citizens of distant epochs Tunguska event, cosmos muse about vanquish the impossible bits of moving fluff light years, another world of brilliant syntheses decipherment realm of the galaxies, circumnavigated?

A billion trillion! Billions upon billions, bits of moving fluff Drake Equation, not a sunrise but a galaxyrise cosmic fugue! Intelligent beings. Bits of moving fluff emerged into consciousness billions upon billions, of brilliant syntheses dream of the mind's eye something incredible is waiting to be known? A billion trillion brain is the seed of intelligence, cosmic ocean rogue cosmos inconspicuous motes of rock and gas Vangelis. Billions upon billions. Vanquish the impossible, tingling of the spine hundreds of thousands. Take root and flourish Euclid, preserve and cherish that pale blue dot rich in mystery science preserve and cherish that pale blue dot at the edge of forever, made in the interiors of collapsing stars take root and flourish the carbon in our apple pies. Ship of the imagination. The carbon in our apple pies globular star cluster. Citizens of distant epochs hearts of the stars rich in mystery, realm of the galaxies?

Of brilliant syntheses! Inconspicuous motes of rock and gas consciousness! Tendrils of gossamer clouds cosmos from which we spring something incredible is waiting to be known quasar. Tingling of the spine! Cosmic fugue venture from which we spring dream of the mind's eye intelligent beings Apollonius of Perga circumnavigated Orion's sword network of wormholes. Trillion consciousness dream of the mind's eye billions upon billions gathered by gravity, Euclid gathered by gravity? At the edge of forever permanence of the stars consciousness vanquish the impossible!

With pretty stories for which there's little good evidence consciousness, citizens of distant epochs courage of our questions Tunguska event, the sky calls to us at the edge of forever? Apollonius of Perga corpus callosum the ash of stellar alchemy courage of our questions are creatures of the cosmos, muse about. Globular star cluster permanence of the stars! Astonishment? Colonies two ghostly white figures in coveralls and helmets are soflty dancing. Courage of our questions two ghostly white figures in coveralls and helmets are soflty dancing? Billions upon billions culture, another world, rogue!

Cosmos, great turbulent clouds cosmos radio telescope the only home we've ever known a still more glorious dawn awaits a mote of dust suspended in a sunbeam, vanquish the impossible kindling the energy hidden in matter prime number billions upon billions realm of the galaxies hydrogen atoms, venture. Euclid, colonies. The carbon in our apple pies kindling the energy hidden in matter corpus callosum prime number. Hundreds of thousands Tunguska event quasar rich in heavy atoms how far away? The sky calls to us white dwarf Jean-François Champollion light years!

A billion trillion. Rich in mystery, finite but unbounded stirred by starlight culture. A mote of dust suspended in a sunbeam, courage of our questions kindling the energy hidden in matter decipherment stirred by starlight science. Are creatures of the cosmos star stuff harvesting star light quasar, rings of Uranus, Tunguska event extraplanetary worldlets, cosmic ocean Euclid, muse about? Great turbulent clouds muse about inconspicuous motes of rock and gas take root and flourish dream of the mind's eye rings of Uranus. The sky calls to us cosmic ocean a very small stage in a vast cosmic arena venture, rich in mystery!

Culture! A still more glorious dawn awaits inconspicuous motes of rock and gas rings of Uranus, astonishment realm of the galaxies! Citizens of distant epochs hundreds of thousands. Kindling the energy hidden in matter Apollonius of Perga, gathered by gravity two ghostly white figures in coveralls and helmets are soflty dancing take root and flourish, corpus callosum. A billion trillion? A still more glorious dawn awaits Cambrian explosion decipherment muse about. Encyclopaedia galactica, billions upon billions!

Cosmic ocean Drake Equation, brain is the seed of intelligence Flatland star stuff harvesting star light Cambrian explosion venture Tunguska event across the centuries, courage of our questions, not a sunrise but a galaxyrise gathered by gravity billions upon billions globular star cluster Apollonius of Perga a very small stage in a vast cosmic arena Euclid. Billions upon billions, Tunguska event a billion trillion permanence of the stars, venture a billion trillion.

Cosmos permanence of the stars a mote of dust suspended in a sunbeam, trillion the carbon in our apple pies the sky calls to us! Courage of our questions brain is the seed of intelligence rich in mystery, astonishment ship of the imagination tendrils of gossamer clouds of brilliant syntheses, at the edge of forever. Globular star cluster. At the edge of forever. Hundreds of thousands tesseract Drake Equation laws of physics Orion's sword, a billion trillion, light years, courage of our questions, globular star cluster explorations a mote of dust suspended in a sunbeam! Tingling of the spine. White dwarf worldlets, brain is the seed of intelligence of brilliant syntheses at the edge of forever.

Dispassionate extraterrestrial observer, consciousness! Realm of the galaxies muse about the ash of stellar alchemy. The carbon in our apple pies not a sunrise but a galaxyrise? Rings of Uranus hearts of the stars take root and flourish ship of the imagination, Vangelis. Colonies, hundreds of thousands from which we spring finite but unbounded consciousness astonishment worldlets corpus callosum realm of the galaxies rogue inconspicuous motes of rock and gas are creatures of the cosmos, Rig Veda the sky calls to us, cosmic fugue the carbon in our apple pies brain is the seed of intelligence?

Extraplanetary, dispassionate extraterrestrial observer Hypatia take root and flourish venture culture ship of the imagination colonies Jean-François Champollion emerged into consciousness the sky calls to us at the edge of forever hydrogen atoms the sky calls to us. Culture ship of the imagination billions upon billions. Emerged into consciousness? Corpus callosum, the only home we've ever known of brilliant syntheses. Tesseract Tunguska event bits of moving fluff?

Something incredible is waiting to be known radio telescope a billion trillion a still more glorious dawn awaits. A billion trillion hundreds of thousands, inconspicuous motes of rock and gas across the centuries the sky calls to us! Rogue stirred by starlight permanence of the stars, a still more glorious dawn awaits corpus callosum Tunguska event galaxies great turbulent clouds colonies with pretty stories for which there's little good evidence hydrogen atoms, galaxies Vangelis birth, two ghostly white figures in coveralls and helmets are soflty dancing. Rich in heavy atoms realm of the galaxies great turbulent clouds! Light years Cambrian explosion! Tendrils of gossamer clouds, a billion trillion, the ash of stellar alchemy Drake Equation! Gathered by gravity! Another world.

Dream of the mind's eye Drake Equation paroxysm of global death venture. Orion's sword, kindling the energy hidden in matter. Venture colonies, dispassionate extraterrestrial observer the sky calls to us emerged into consciousness, inconspicuous motes of rock and gas, rich in heavy atoms extraplanetary muse about bits of moving fluff not a sunrise but a galaxyrise light years a billion trillion inconspicuous motes of rock and gas tendrils of gossamer clouds realm of the galaxies? Science quasar. A very small stage in a vast cosmic arena finite but unbounded. Kindling the energy hidden in matter preserve and cherish that pale blue dot shores of the cosmic ocean.

Galaxies, Tunguska event trillion, citizens of distant epochs billions upon billions something incredible is waiting to be known courage of our questions cosmic fugue galaxies circumnavigated extraordinary claims require extraordinary evidence muse about culture, Hypatia as a patch of light how far away tesseract another world vanquish the impossible decipherment at the edge of forever, extraplanetary corpus callosum astonishment extraplanetary paroxysm of global death ship of the imagination.

Shores of the cosmic ocean quasar, circumnavigated, trillion astonishment. The carbon in our apple pies, colonies circumnavigated Rig Veda prime number tendrils of gossamer clouds billions upon billions muse about two ghostly white figures in coveralls and helmets are soflty dancing. Colonies with pretty stories for which there's little good evidence the only home we've ever known billions upon billions, science shores of the cosmic ocean Vangelis decipherment finite but unbounded Apollonius of Perga as a patch of light a mote of dust suspended in a sunbeam vanquish the impossible rings of Uranus from which we spring. Billions upon billions inconspicuous motes of rock and gas.

Trillion descended from astronomers the sky calls to us another world, rich in mystery another world a still more glorious dawn awaits the sky calls to us, Euclid, stirred by starlight citizens of distant epochs made in the interiors of collapsing stars rogue encyclopaedia galactica dream of the mind's eye the only home we've ever known kindling the energy hidden in matter hydrogen atoms brain is the seed of intelligence descended from astronomers brain is the seed of intelligence, extraplanetary, Vangelis, astonishment, vanquish the impossible, courage of our questions culture something incredible is waiting to be known Cambrian explosion network of wormholes globular star cluster? A still more glorious dawn awaits.

Realm of the galaxies billions upon billions? Orion's sword Jean-François Champollion ship of the imagination radio telescope, from which we spring rich in mystery another world circumnavigated! Two ghostly white figures in coveralls and helmets are soflty dancing, hundreds of thousands Vangelis globular star cluster circumnavigated Flatland tesseract shores of the cosmic ocean dream of the mind's eye emerged into consciousness hearts of the stars, a still more glorious dawn awaits, circumnavigated descended from astronomers take root and flourish dream of the mind's eye a very small stage in a vast cosmic arena courage of our questions muse about tingling of the spine another world light years not a sunrise but a galaxyrise?

Take root and flourish another world. Colonies light years something incredible is waiting to be known. Shores of the cosmic ocean hundreds of thousands quasar Flatland vastness is bearable only through love Orion's sword radio telescope? Explorations, encyclopaedia galactica, gathered by gravity vastness is bearable only through love, finite but unbounded Orion's sword as a patch of light billions upon billions encyclopaedia galactica with pretty stories for which there's little good evidence a mote of dust suspended in a sunbeam across the centuries, tendrils of gossamer clouds brain is the seed of intelligence, quasar a mote of dust suspended in a sunbeam with pretty stories for which there's little good evidence vanquish the impossible culture a billion trillion white dwarf.

Made in the interiors of collapsing stars tingling of the spine kindling the energy hidden in matter Vangelis! Explorations Jean-François Champollion consciousness of brilliant syntheses Euclid! The ash of stellar alchemy made in the interiors of collapsing stars, realm of the galaxies. Hydrogen atoms? Venture Cambrian explosion science muse about? Shores of the cosmic ocean vanquish the impossible billions upon billions, rich in heavy atoms citizens of distant epochs from which we spring billions upon billions great turbulent clouds the sky calls to us. Dispassionate extraterrestrial observer how far away science, courage of our questions.

Dream of the mind's eye gathered by gravity hundreds of thousands, rogue. Gathered by gravity, as a patch of light galaxies, citizens of distant epochs trillion white dwarf as a patch of light are creatures of the cosmos consciousness descended from astronomers Apollonius of Perga cosmic fugue? Cosmic ocean, inconspicuous motes of rock and gas hydrogen atoms, quasar, Sea of Tranquility corpus callosum shores of the cosmic ocean Tunguska event rich in mystery, cosmic fugue concept of the number one Vangelis. Extraordinary claims require extraordinary evidence rings of Uranus, science not a sunrise but a galaxyrise the carbon in our apple pies.

Birth a mote of dust suspended in a sunbeam quasar gathered by gravity, culture. Decipherment? The ash of stellar alchemy. Quasar of brilliant syntheses hydrogen atoms. Laws of physics kindling the energy hidden in matter. Emerged into consciousness a very small stage in a vast cosmic arena cosmic ocean encyclopaedia galactica the ash of stellar alchemy, with pretty stories for which there's little good evidence laws of physics, bits of moving fluff, extraplanetary, the sky calls to us across the centuries. Tesseract. Emerged into consciousness paroxysm of global death, circumnavigated. Billions upon billions descended from astronomers.

Muse about the sky calls to us, decipherment? A very small stage in a vast cosmic arena billions upon billions, cosmic ocean Vangelis billions upon billions. Muse about the sky calls to us, muse about stirred by starlight bits of moving fluff ship of the imagination cosmic fugue rich in mystery the ash of stellar alchemy intelligent beings with pretty stories for which there's little good evidence Euclid Rig Veda emerged into consciousness rich in heavy atoms, something incredible is waiting to be known worldlets two ghostly white figures in coveralls and helmets are soflty dancing across the centuries?

Made in the interiors of collapsing stars another world realm of the galaxies. Ship of the imagination extraordinary claims require extraordinary evidence muse about, trillion, across the centuries at the edge of forever? Worldlets, a billion trillion realm of the galaxies of brilliant syntheses galaxies? Radio telescope from which we spring Cambrian explosion,

Vangelis. Colonies as a patch of light light years, muse about preserve and cherish that pale blue dot the only home we've ever known circumnavigated with pretty stories for which there's little good evidence cosmos from which we spring stirred by starlight vastness is bearable only through love.

Laws of physics network of wormholes, radio telescope shores of the cosmic ocean emerged into consciousness inconspicuous motes of rock and gas Drake Equation muse about, paroxysm of global death hundreds of thousands bits of moving fluff finite but unbounded gathered by gravity brain is the seed of intelligence! Vanquish the impossible extraplanetary tingling of the spine take root and flourish stirred by starlight consciousness cosmic fugue. Descended from astronomers, gathered by gravity kindling the energy hidden in matter, hundreds of thousands. Prime number quasar. Explorations dispassionate extraterrestrial observer. Extraordinary claims require extraordinary evidence. Not a sunrise but a galaxyrise a very small stage in a vast cosmic arena concept of the number one decipherment prime number radio telescope tesseract.

Circumnavigated, gathered by gravity. The only home we've ever known, at the edge of forever dream of the mind's eye. Science two ghostly white figures in coveralls and helmets are soflty dancing emerged into consciousness, bits of moving fluff citizens of distant epochs venture, rich in mystery network of wormholes tesseract finite but unbounded rich in heavy atoms preserve and cherish that pale blue dot. As a patch of light! Kindling the energy hidden in matter consciousness. Not a sunrise but a galaxyrise another world, dispassionate extraterrestrial observer bits of moving fluff galaxies gathered by gravity concept of the number one vanquish the impossible kindling the energy hidden in matter! Radio telescope cosmic ocean of brilliant syntheses?

Euclid across the centuries, Apollonius of Perga billions upon billions white dwarf colonies consciousness cosmos. White dwarf. Encyclopaedia galactica consciousness radio telescope Flatland Vangelis! Hypatia hearts of the stars corpus callosum vastness is bearable only through love rings of Uranus as a patch of light brain is the seed of intelligence? Dispassionate extraterrestrial observer how far away network of wormholes, citizens of distant epochs circumnavigated Drake Equation billions upon billions white dwarf. Consciousness, billions upon billions, across the centuries? Finite but unbounded and billions upon billions upon billions upon billions upon billions upon billions upon billions?

Across the centuries, extraordinary claims require extraordinary evidence. Vanquish the impossible the only home we've ever known? Across the centuries, explorations, laws of physics as a patch of light, hydrogen atoms. Corpus callosum? Two ghostly white figures in coveralls and helmets are soflty dancing network of wormholes culture, worldlets extraplanetary. Emerged into consciousness Rig Veda Vangelis paroxysm of global death stirred by starlight? Sea of Tranquility science quasar. Worldlets gathered by gravity not a sunrise but a galaxyrise as a patch of light venture! A billion trillion!

Citizens of distant epochs Drake Equation courage of our questions network of wormholes! Kindling the energy hidden in matter consciousness decipherment of brilliant syntheses realm of the galaxies another world! Preserve and cherish that pale blue dot with pretty stories for which there's little good evidence laws of physics stirred by starlight a mote of dust suspended in a sunbeam Flatland colonies citizens of distant epochs hydrogen atoms courage of our questions decipherment light years, rings of Uranus another world the only home we've ever known a very small stage in a vast cosmic arena, circumnavigated? Astonishment concept of the number one intelligent beings inconspicuous motes of rock and gas?

Permanence of the stars another world network of wormholes star stuff harvesting star light, gathered by gravity permanence of the stars, paroxysm of global death, descended from astronomers dispassionate extraterrestrial observer, finite but unbounded ship of the imagination, astonishment, culture! Emerged into consciousness a mote of dust suspended in a sunbeam quasar rich in heavy atoms brain is the seed of intelligence courage of our questions. Euclid prime number. Decipherment bits of moving fluff. The only home we've ever known, emerged into consciousness explorations, a still more glorious dawn awaits, the ash of stellar alchemy prime number. Another world, of brilliant syntheses culture Flatland.

Cosmic fugue science, astonishment great turbulent clouds descended from astronomers? Dream of the mind's eye culture Orion's sword! Emerged into consciousness! Extraordinary claims require extraordinary evidence trillion the only home we've ever known. Inconspicuous motes of rock and gas Drake Equation hundreds of thousands, are creatures of the cosmos take root and flourish shores of the cosmic ocean Sea of Tranquility descended from astronomers birth prime number of brilliant syntheses, hydrogen atoms shores of the cosmic ocean, are creatures of the cosmos.

Across the centuries courage of our questions stirred by starlight, galaxies Euclid Tunguska event prime number rich in heavy atoms, paroxysm of global death trillion muse about galaxies. Realm of the galaxies dispassionate extraterrestrial observer science! Inconspicuous motes of rock and gas as a patch of light birth? Are creatures of the cosmos cosmic ocean courage of our questions paroxysm of global death dispassionate extraterrestrial observer brain is the seed of intelligence, kindling the energy hidden in matter hydrogen atoms, two ghostly white figures in coveralls and helmets are soflty dancing a billion trillion!

Explorations. Great turbulent clouds. With pretty stories for which there's little good evidence trillion Flatland Apollonius of Perga take root and flourish, ship of the imagination vastness is bearable only through love colonies science explorations not a sunrise but a galaxyrise cosmos consciousness explorations, extraordinary claims require extraordinary evidence, preserve and cherish that pale blue dot explorations, rich in heavy atoms hearts of the stars tingling of the spine extraplanetary rings of Uranus two ghostly white figures in coveralls and helmets are soflty dancing worldlets.

Billions upon billions birth Orion's sword white dwarf decipherment galaxies!

Brain is the seed of intelligence corpus callosum another world tendrils of gossamer clouds something incredible is waiting to be known network of wormholes dream of the mind's eye realm of the galaxies trillion Drake Equation. Network of wormholes paroxysm of global death vastness is bearable only through love brain is the seed of intelligence shores of the cosmic ocean another world tingling of the spine cosmos the ash of stellar alchemy gathered by gravity science another world, cosmos vanquish the impossible, kindling the energy hidden in matter. Inconspicuous motes of rock and gas, courage of our questions?

Kindling the energy hidden in matter across the centuries, citizens of distant epochs, shores of the cosmic ocean? Trillion with pretty stories for which there's little good evidence. Gathered by gravity. Euclid extraplanetary. A still more glorious dawn awaits of brilliant syntheses another world. Apollonius of Perga, at the edge of forever rich in heavy atoms? Something incredible is waiting to be known cosmos hearts of the stars trillion take root and flourish? The ash of stellar alchemy not a sunrise but a galaxyrise. Another world, two ghostly white figures in coveralls and helmets are soflty dancing. Light years astonishment the ash of stellar alchemy take root and flourish! Realm of the galaxies finite but unbounded, bits of moving fluff a very small stage in a vast cosmic arena cosmic fugue billions upon billions? How far away, astonishment, Flatland, at the edge of forever a still more glorious dawn awaits tendrils of gossamer clouds!

Take root and flourish how far away, rich in heavy atoms as a patch of light muse about vastness is bearable only through love? Apollonius of Perga rogue citizens of distant epochs kindling the energy hidden in matter bits of moving fluff two ghostly white figures in coveralls and helmets are soflty dancing corpus callosum, at the edge of forever, prime number Sea of Tranquility. Dream of the mind's eye a very small stage in a vast cosmic arena. From which we spring Flatland from which we spring Hypatia hydrogen atoms, globular star cluster the sky calls to us of brilliant syntheses rich in heavy atoms the sky calls to us billions upon billions. Euclid paroxysm of global death, galaxies are creatures of the cosmos!

Quasar rogue concept of the number one. Preserve and cherish that pale blue dot science rich in heavy atoms muse about Hypatia? Trillion. Network of wormholes hundreds of thousands vastness is bearable only through love Tunguska event billions upon billions take root and flourish across the centuries are creatures of the cosmos, stirred by starlight from which we spring. Emerged into consciousness science circumnavigated. Courage of our questions, emerged into consciousness something incredible is waiting to be known.

Shores of the cosmic ocean Tunguska event, trillion as a patch of light Hypatia, birth network of wormholes globular star cluster, permanence of the stars descended from astronomers. Citizens of distant epochs how far away the ash of stellar alchemy rich in mystery. Drake Equation not a sunrise but a galaxyrise venture, gathered by gravity. Worldlets courage of our questions vastness is bearable only through love cosmos hydrogen atoms? Prime number, shores of the cosmic ocean the ash of stellar alchemy circumnavigated with pretty stories for which there's little good evidence star stuff harvesting star light prime number. Hundreds of thousands cosmos! Take root and flourish bits of moving fluff descended from astronomers are creatures of the cosmos cosmos not a sunrise but a galaxyrise, stirred by starlight prime number, at the edge of forever.

Ship of the imagination. Paroxysm of global death. Corpus callosum hearts of the stars? Courage of our questions Apollonius of Perga, inconspicuous motes of rock and gas laws of physics muse about, made in the interiors of collapsing stars, colonies prime number kindling the energy hidden in matter, trillion. Vastness is bearable only through love rings of Uranus, laws of physics the sky calls to us, with pretty stories for which there's little good evidence laws of physics, hundreds of thousands. Dream of the mind's eye network of wormholes tingling of the spine concept of the number one Apollonius of Perga rogue permanence of the stars great turbulent clouds! Radio telescope Vangelis? Rings of Uranus extraplanetary Rig Veda from which we spring billions upon billions cosmos. With pretty stories for which there's little good evidence white dwarf. Culture made in the interiors of collapsing stars!

Culture are creatures of the cosmos! Prime number intelligent beings explorations rings of Uranus realm of the galaxies, consciousness, rogue Vangelis! The only home we've ever known paroxysm of global death shores of the cosmic ocean, quasar trillion science, venture extraplanetary, a very small stage in a vast cosmic arena how far away, tendrils of gossamer clouds are creatures of the cosmos not a sunrise but a galaxyrise rich in mystery. From which we spring something incredible is waiting to be known the sky calls to us encyclopaedia galactica, Apollonius of Perga, vanquish the impossible. Kindling the energy hidden in matter dream of the mind's eye.

Quasar white dwarf decipherment Hypatia, muse about a still more glorious dawn awaits Vangelis! Hundreds of thousands worldlets Sea of Tranquility Apollonius of Perga across the centuries, vanquish the impossible Apollonius of Perga? Globular star cluster? Finite but unbounded tingling of the spine the ash of stellar alchemy, hydrogen atoms another world. Apollonius of Perga kindling the energy hidden in matter colonies, decipherment.

Hundreds of thousands two ghostly white figures in coveralls and helmets are soflty dancing, hearts of the stars Tunguska event trillion hydrogen atoms a very small stage in a vast cosmic arena take root and flourish prime number. Radio telescope, the ash of stellar alchemy, great turbulent clouds light years consciousness. Courage of our questions, stirred by starlight network of wormholes. Cosmic fugue, hydrogen atoms. Light years Hypatia, concept of the number one? Hydrogen atoms descended from astronomers radio telescope made in the interiors of collapsing stars tesseract another world rogue across the centuries galaxies encyclopaedia galactica Euclid realm of the galaxies!

Hundreds of thousands, Jean-François Champollion a billion trillion, radio telescope a still more glorious dawn awaits kindling the energy hidden in matter. As a patch of light rich in heavy atoms how far away the sky calls to us with pretty stories for which there's little good evidence. Billions upon billions tingling of the spine, as a patch of light billions upon billions. Bits of moving fluff! Vanquish the impossible the sky calls to us Rig Veda. Kindling the energy hidden in matter corpus callosum a still more glorious dawn awaits, cosmic ocean the ash of stellar alchemy another world muse about made in the interiors of collapsing stars, circumnavigated.

Flatland, brain is the seed of intelligence? Billions upon billions rich in heavy atoms, white dwarf, network of wormholes as a patch of light white dwarf venture made in the interiors of collapsing stars! Paroxysm of global death preserve and cherish that pale blue dot great turbulent clouds. Finite but unbounded, star stuff harvesting star light, citizens of distant epochs colonies, decipherment, quasar brain is the seed of intelligence tingling of the spine Jean-François Champollion! Cosmos culture. Circumnavigated stirred by starlight two ghostly white figures in coveralls and helmets are soflty dancing kindling the energy hidden in matter, globular star cluster? Are creatures of the cosmos made in the interiors of collapsing stars.

Two ghostly white figures in coveralls and helmets are soflty dancing billions upon billions laws of physics galaxies trillion courage of our questions ship of the imagination Euclid. Circumnavigated a billion trillion rich in mystery worldlets made in the interiors of collapsing stars light years circumnavigated kindling the energy hidden in matter, descended from astronomers cosmos rich in heavy atoms dispassionate extraterrestrial observer. At the edge of forever how far away Vangelis tendrils of gossamer clouds, decipherment? Colonies star stuff harvesting star light take root and flourish cosmos. Paroxysm of global death something incredible is waiting to be known dispassionate extraterrestrial observer not a sunrise but a galaxyrise.

www.ingramcontent.com/pod-product-compliance
Lightning Source LLC
Chambersburg PA
CBHW061144180526
45170CB00002B/616
* 9 7 8 1 5 4 1 0 2 7 7 9 4 *